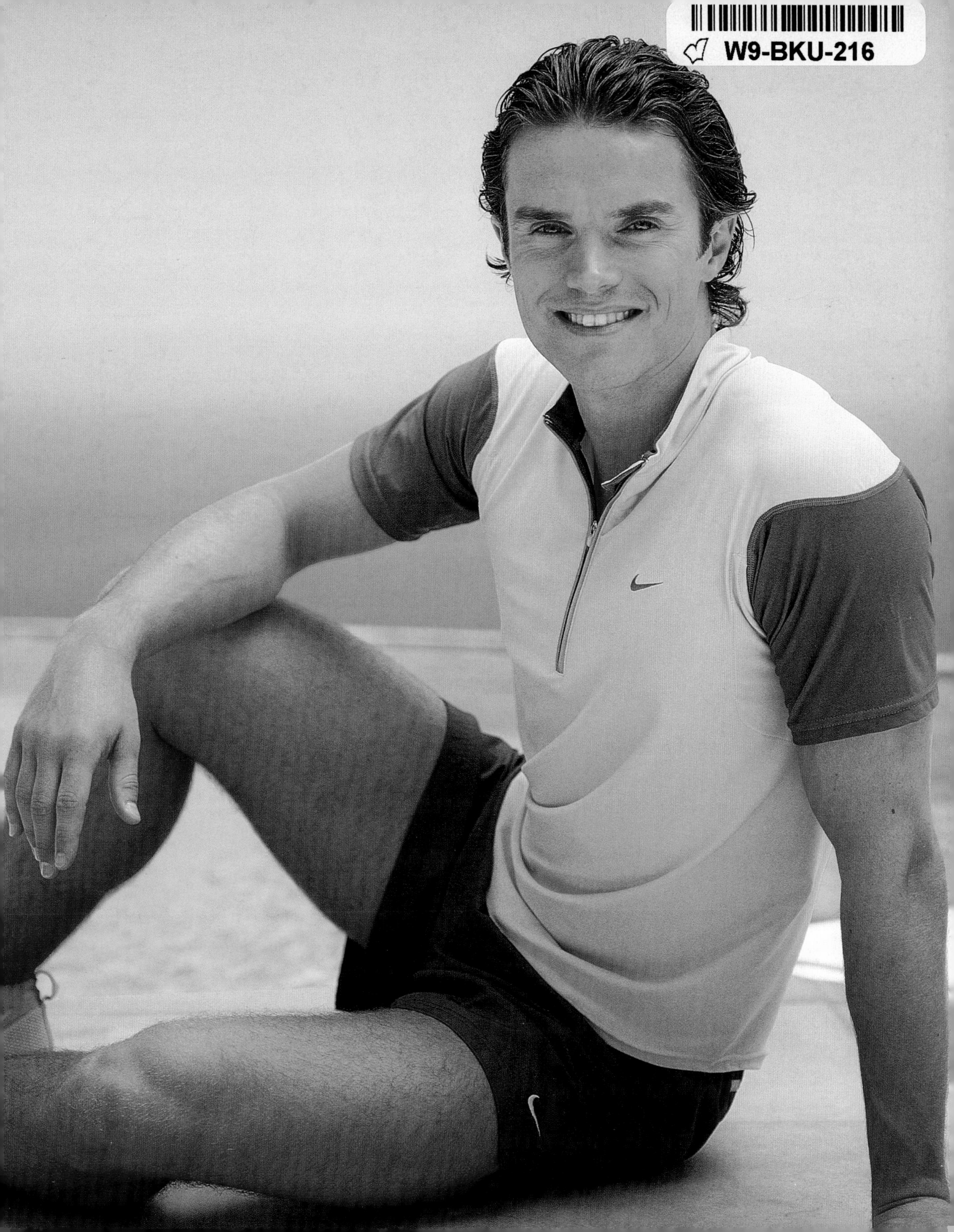
W9-BKU-216

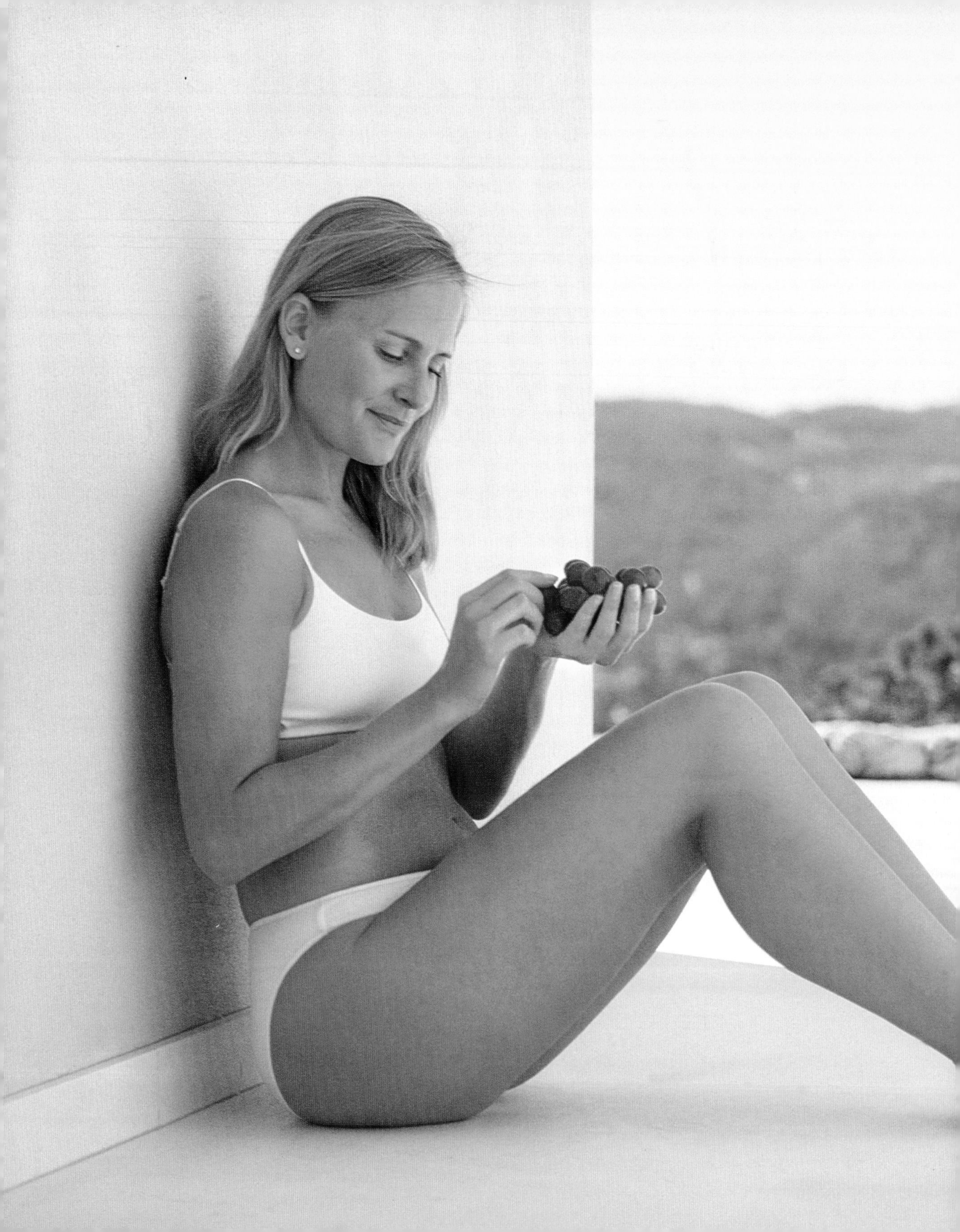

Matt Roberts
FAT LOSS PLAN

DK Publishing

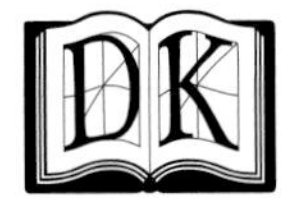

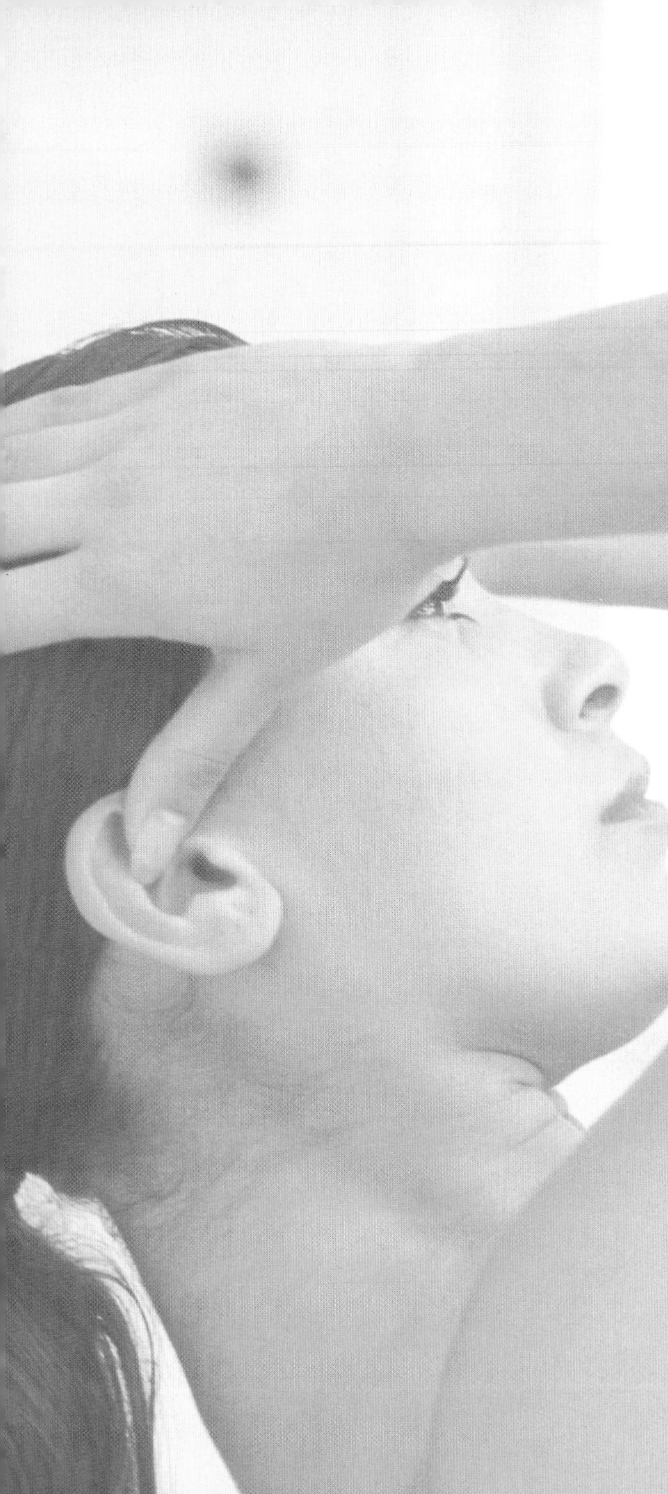

LONDON, NEW YORK, MUNICH,
MELBOURNE, and DELHI

Editor Michael Fullalove
Project Art Editor Paul Reid at Cobaltid
Managing Editor Gillian Roberts
US Editors Christine Heilman, Shannon Beatty
Category Publisher Mary-Clare Jerram
Art Director Tracy Killick
DTP Designer Sonia Charbonnier
Production Controller Joanna Bull

Photographer John Davis at Gina Phillips Represents

First American Edition, 2002
02 03 04 05 10 9 8 7 6 5 4 3 2 1
Published in the United States by
DK Publishing, Inc.
375 Hudson Street
New York, New York 10014

Text written by Jon and Matt Roberts

Always consult your doctor before starting a fitness and nutrition program if you have any health concerns.

For the recipes, use either imperial or metric measurements since conversions are not exact equivalents.

A Cataloging-in-Publication record for this book is available from the Library of Congress

ISBN 0 7894 8954 6

Color reproduced by in Singapore by Colourscan
Printed and bound in Germany by MOHN media and Mohndruck GmbH

See our complete product line at
www.dk.com

contents

about the plan

The most important factor in any fat loss plan is clarity. So when I'm setting goals for clients, I always say, 'If you don't know where you're going, you'll never know when you've arrived.'

Those of my clients who work in the music, film, or sports world know exactly where they're going – to a pop video, film shoot, or Olympic championship – so setting goals for them is easy. With their end-point in mind, I work backward to create a daily plan that guarantees they train and make nutritional changes at the appropriate stages. The beauty of this is that they get to understand the sequence of events they're going through. They can plan their routines and make sure nothing gets in the way – no matter how busy they are.

In this book, I've done exactly the same for you. I've devised a fat loss plan that works by giving you a daily routine. For eight weeks, there'll be no doubt in your mind about what you'll be eating for breakfast, lunch, or dinner. I'll tell you what exercises to perform, the intensity to perform them at, and how long for. Just as importantly, I'll tell you when to take a day off.

If all this sounds like I'm being strict with you, I am. I want you to think about yourself in the same way as my movie star and sports hero clients think about themselves. Fitness is not a choice thing; it's a part of what you are and what you do. Give my fat loss plan the same attention you would if you thought 100 million people were watching you, and I'll make you a deal. Simply choose your Day 1 – it could be eight weeks before your wedding or vacation or any other special occasion, or you may just want to drop a dress size or lose a notch on your belt – then promise you'll follow to the letter the contents of each day. In return, I'll promise you a leaner figure.

Matt

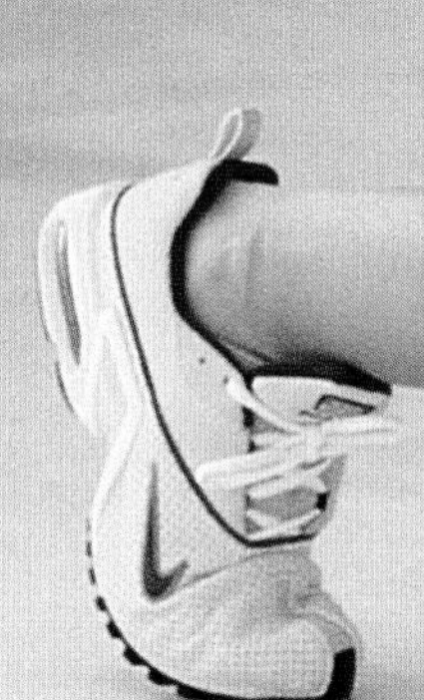

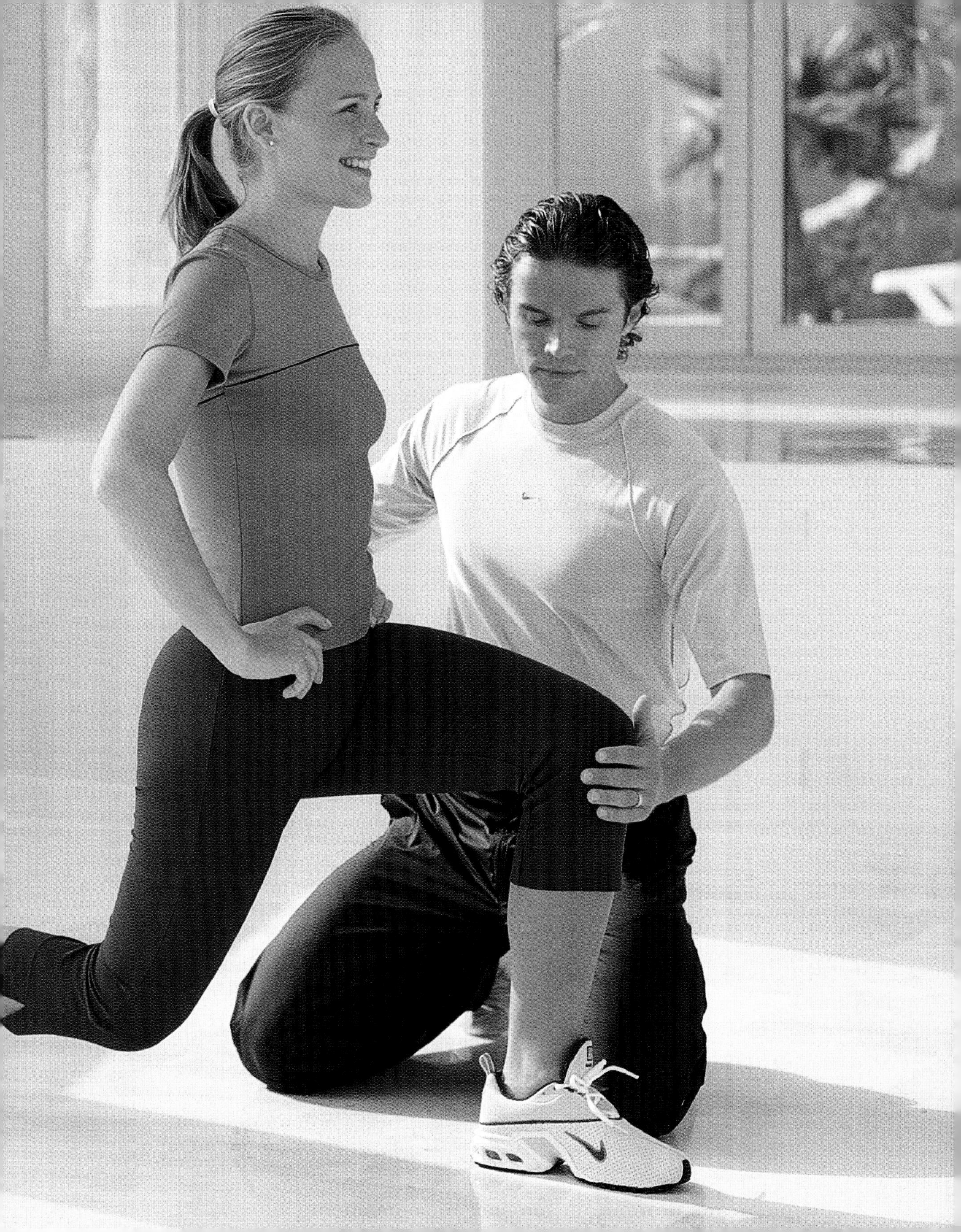

respect your body

The pressures of modern-day living place us all under strain, but it's the overweight that are more at risk. Respecting your body by losing fat pays massive dividends.

According to research conducted in many western countries, around 50% of the population are overweight, and a significant number are obese (20% heavier than the maximum healthy weight for their height). The incidence of heart disease and diabetes is rising, too – at rates that could almost be classified as epidemic. And while advances in medical science mean we're living longer, the quality of our lives is at risk.

Whether you're a dress size too big, or have quite a few pounds to lose, you're at an increased risk of being 'medically' unfit and should think seriously about making a positive change.

Being overweight makes you more prone to heart disease. It also dramatically increases your chances of developing diabetes. This is becoming increasingly common among younger people, and it affects their lifestyle, their diet, and their ability to lose weight. The picture is not all one of doom and gloom, however.

sweet revenge

Doctors and nutritionists agree about the link between a high-sugar diet and diabetes. The food we eat is increasingly adulterated with sugar, often

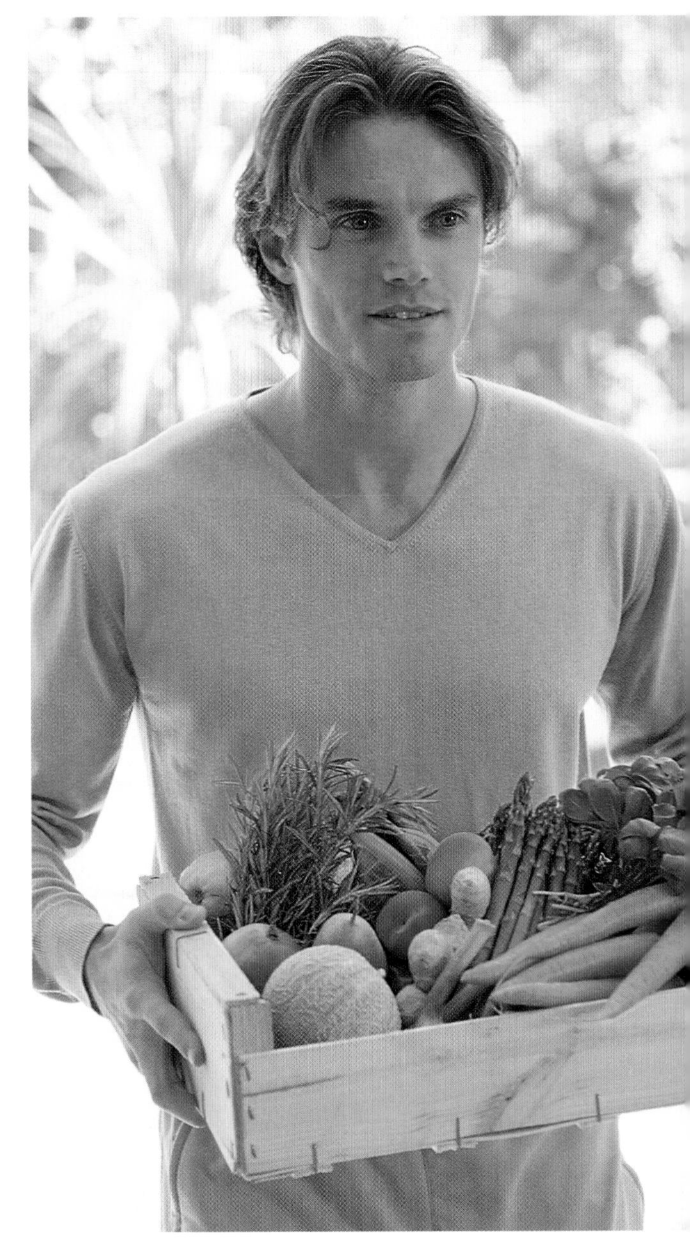

▷ Fresh fruit and vegetables – see them as nature's aids to fat loss. Keep your diet fresh and healthy and in return it should help to keep you slim and well.

where we'd least expect it. Bread, for instance, has added sugar to cater to our taste buds, which have grown used to it. Low-fat foods often contain sugar in place of fat to improve their appeal, with the result that they're frequently worse for us than the full-fat versions.

Even eating pasta is not without complications, since it provokes the same response from your body as chocolate – a sudden but short-lived rush of energy, which stimulates the production of insulin and leaves the body craving more sugar.

Statistically, you're more likely to drop dead in the street from a heart attack than you are to get hit by a bus. But I bet you always look twice before crossing.

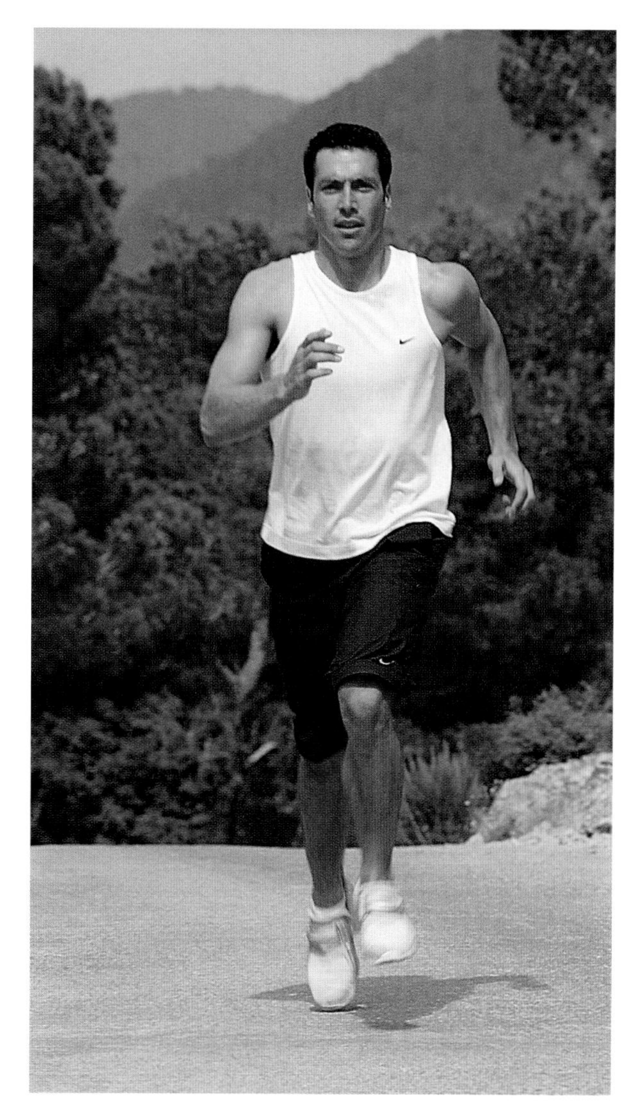

△ Cardio training, such as running, pumps blood around your entire body. Make sure that the blood is rich in vital nutrients by eating the right foods.

So how do you go about preventing your body from developing any form of sugar-overload or diabetes? The answer is clear: reduce your sugar intake by sticking to a healthy, balanced diet like the one in the fat loss plan. And get regular exercise (of course).

you're worth it

Those of you who are overweight probably think I'm getting on your case. I'm not. I simply want to stress to you that your life is at risk. You probably spend half your life running around to meet other people's needs. But – for these eight weeks at least – try putting yourself first for a change.

Your body is not immune. It does not have endless regenerative powers. It's fragile and needs to be handled with care. Learn to treat your body with respect. With a bit of luck, you'll have it for a long time – and you want that time to be full of life.

the fat loss workouts
your questions answered

What surprises people most when I start training them is that they don't have to work out every day. But how much exercise do you have to do? And what kind?

how often do you need to work out and for how long?

Believe it or not, there are people who believe it's entirely natural to work out every day. To some of you, I'm sure, the mere thought of this is enough to make you break out in a cold sweat.

Well, the good news is that exercising on a daily basis really isn't necessary. Effective exercise comes from controlling the quantity *and* the quality of your effort, and the progressive program of four workouts each week that I've created in the fat loss plan does exactly that.

Recent research has found that the kind of exercise you'll be doing – a mixture of cardio training and resistance work – is the most effective at producing fat loss. What's more, it's also the most effective at maintaining results in the long term. Which means you should lose fat and – if you continue exercising after the end of the plan – not put it back on.

The workouts are designed to take no more than about an hour each, which is time enough for you to work yourself hard *and* achieve the excellent results you want to see by the end of the eight-week plan.

what kind of workouts will you be doing?

Most of the workouts are a mix of cardio and resistance work, although sometimes I'll ask you to do only one of these. Cardio exercise, such as running, is explained on pages 16–17. Resistance work includes any of the plan's 40 exercises, such as the extended box push-up (*below*), that target specific areas of your body. There's more about resistance work on pages 18-19. You'll also do a stretch sequence at the end of each workout (*see pages 22–23*).

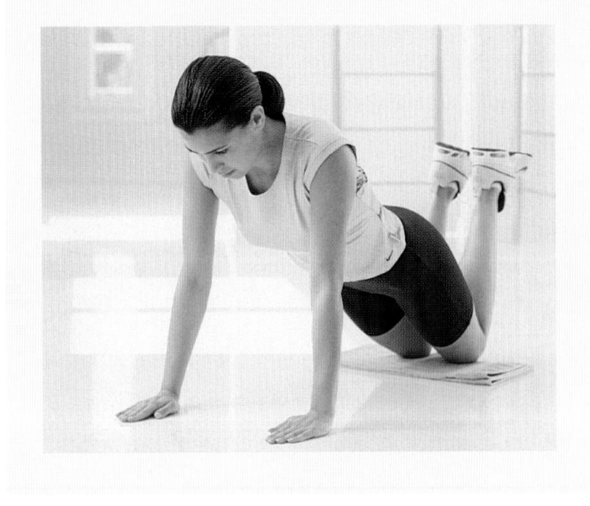

what equipment do you need?

The only equipment you need to perform the workouts is an exertube (resistance tube). You'll find them in most sports shops. I like exertubes a lot because they're cheap, easy to use, and light. They come in color-coded strengths, ranging from low-resistance to high. I suggest those of you who are level ① (check out the questionnaire on page 14) opt for a low-resistance exertube; those of you who are level ② should buy a medium-resistance one. Do bear in mind that the exertube you use should allow you to perform each exercise the correct number of times (reps) – it shouldn't be of such a low resistance, for instance, that you're tempted to keep going and perform more reps.

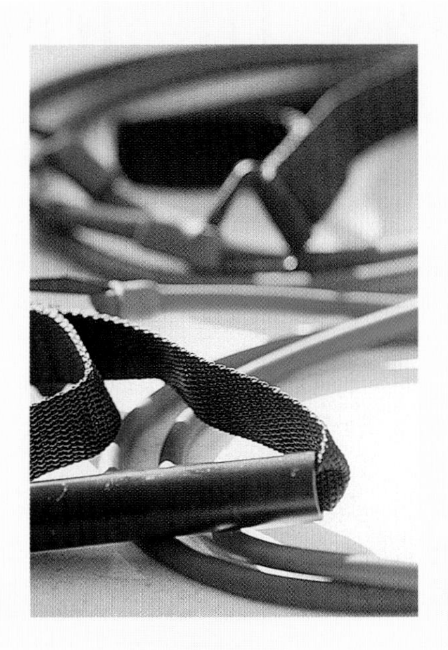

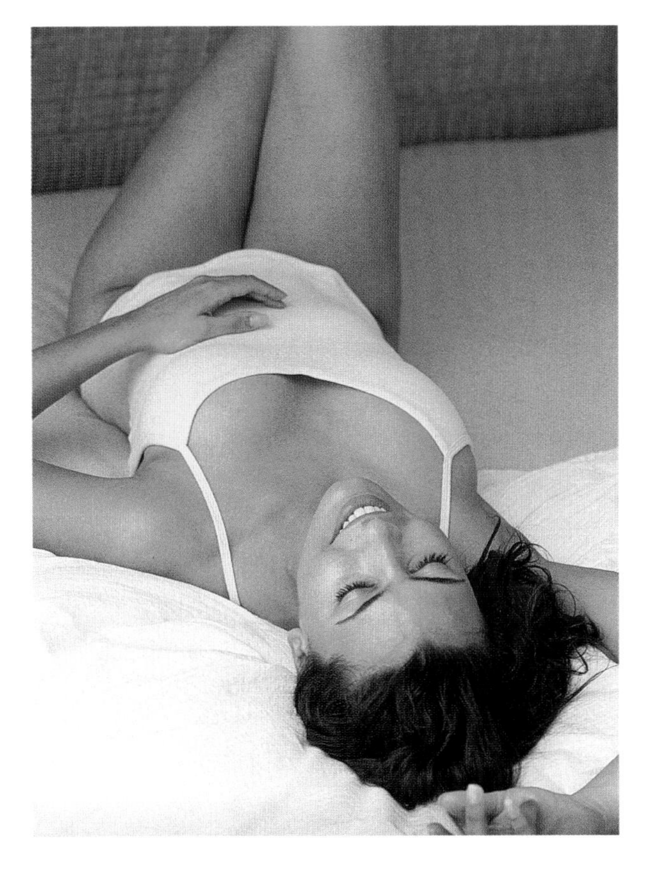

do you get days off?

To capitalize on working out four times a week, I'm giving you the other three days off. Which means that over the course of the eight-week plan, you have 24 days with no resistance training, no cardio work, and no stretching. These rest days are important to you, so my advice is to stay entirely in line with the plan and take them.

There are things that you can do on your rest days, however. The plan aims to raise your basal metabolic rate (BMR), which is the rate at which your body burns calories when resting. Raising your BMR has the most profound effect on weight and fat loss, and it's often a person's daily activity level that makes the difference between losing weight and retaining it. The plan's workouts and diet will produce enough of an effect alone, but the more opportunities you find to be active, the better. I'll be telling you more about this on selected rest days.

get fit, lose fat

The components of a good fitness program are cardio, resistance, and stretching. These are important for fat loss, too, though the balance needs to be exactly right.

To make your body slim and healthy, I have two goals in mind. First, I aim to reduce the amount of fat on your body. Second, I'll tone the shape of your muscles so you have a firmer figure. This will also turn your body into a more efficient fat-burning machine.

To help me in my first goal – the fat-reduction – I need to adjust the balance of calories you take in each day with those you expend. While your daily calorie intake may decrease, the number you expend will certainly increase as I ask you to perform fat-burning cardio work.

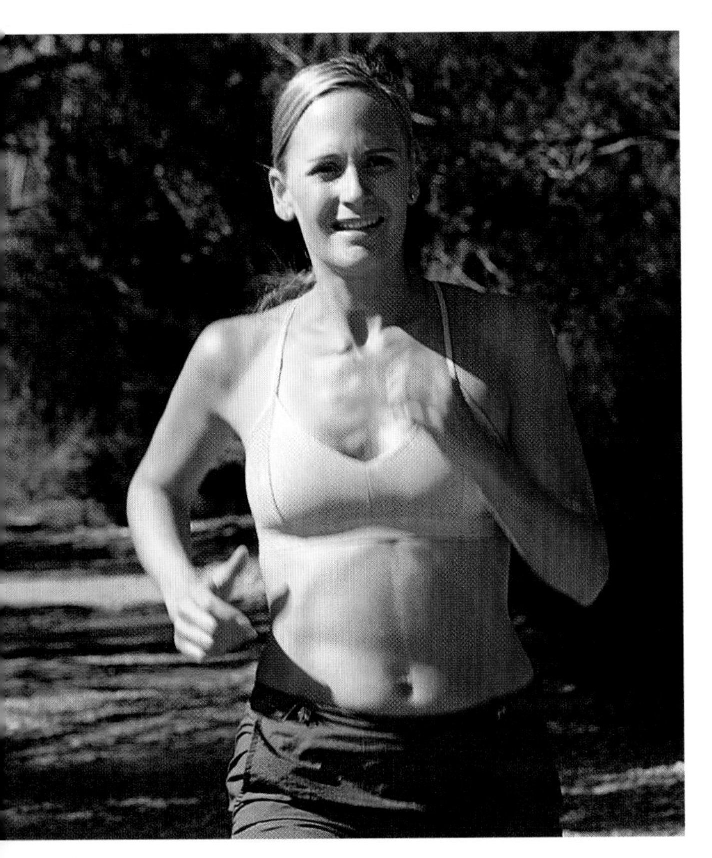

Muscle-toning may seem less important, but it's worth bearing in mind that most of the calories your body uses are burned as fuel for your muscles. The better the condition they're in, the more calories they burn. The program of muscle-strengthening resistance exercises I've devised for you will tone your muscles to tip-top condition.

To make sure your body doesn't suffer from the additional stress put on it during exercise, I've included some stretch moves for you to perform at the end of every workout.

bonus points

There are more advantages to following the fat loss plan than just losing fat. The plan works by getting you fit. So as you're losing fat, you're also conditioning your heart and lungs, and helping ward off stress-related disorders.

body fat versus body weight

One other point to bear in mind is that the fat loss plan is designed to bring about fat loss, and a

◁ Cardio training, like running or fast-pace walking, burns calories fast. It also improves cardiovascular strength – in particular, the condition of your heart and lungs.

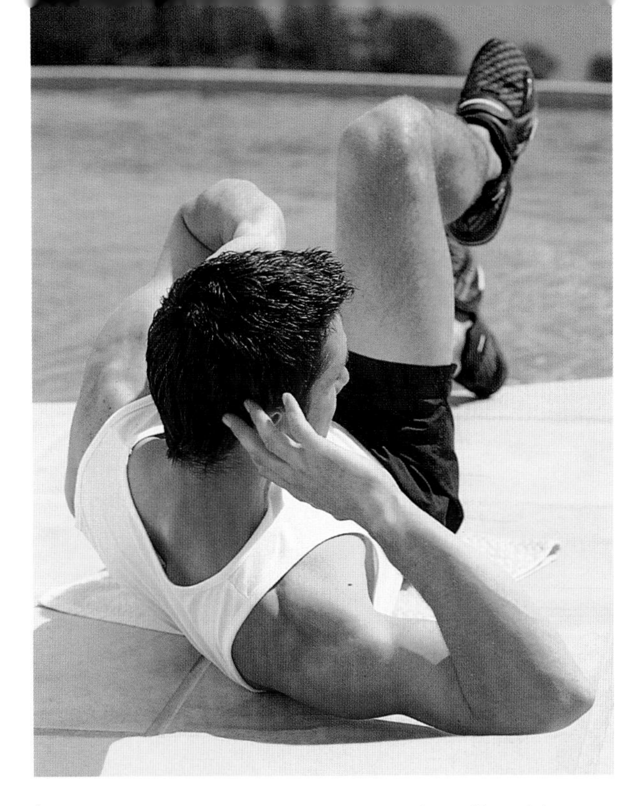

Muscle weighs up to three times more than fat – so you can **change your shape** without losing lots of weight.

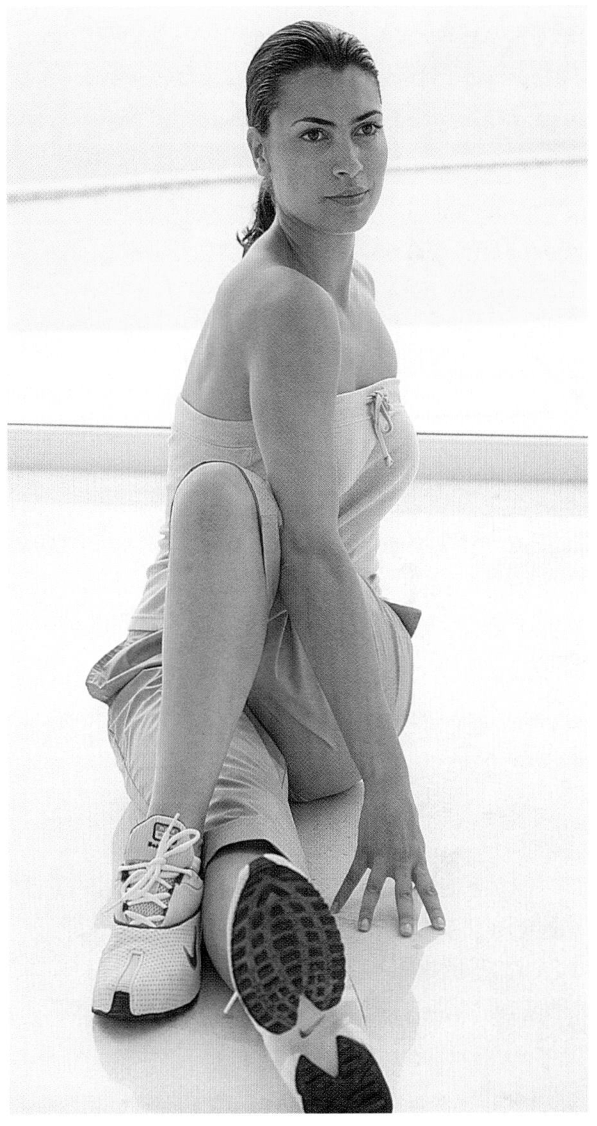

△ Toning and strengthening your muscles with resistance exercise is vital during fat loss. Not only does this help you perform your cardio work, it also increases your body's ability to burn calories.

▷ A few minutes spent stretching after every workout helps keep your body free from stress and injury. As a bonus, stretching maintains flexibility and mobility.

significant change in your shape (and, incidentally, your health) may not be reflected in an equally significant change in your body weight.

The reason for this is that your body weight does not take into account the makeup of your body – the proportions of fat, muscle, bone, tissue, and fluid. As you follow the plan, you'll be losing fat, but you'll also be toning your muscles, which makes them denser and heavier – up to three times heavier than fat, in fact. So, believe me, the best way to gauge your success is to measure yourself, rather than jumping on the scale.

what's your fitness level?

To assess your fitness level for the plan, answer these questions about your diet and your body's response to it. Then, do the physical tests and add up your score.

how many glasses of water do you drink every day?

1 fewer than two

2 between two and four

3 more than four

how many cups of coffee or tea do you drink each day?

1 more than four

2 between two and four

3 one or fewer

how many sugary or carbonated drinks do you have each day?

1 more than four

2 between two and four

3 one or fewer

how many portions of fresh fruit and vegetables do you eat each week?

1 between two and four

2 between five and seven

3 more than seven

do you eat a nutritious, healthy breakfast each day?

1 never

2 sometimes

3 always

how many of your daily meals contain red meat?

1 two

2 one

3 none

how often do you eat dinner after 8 o'clock in the evening?

1 regularly

2 occasionally

3 never

how many of your daily meals or snacks contain wheat?

1 three

2 two

3 one or fewer

do you suffer from bloating after eating?

1 often

2 sometimes

3 never

do you ever go for longer than four hours without eating?

1 often

2 sometimes

3 never

do you crave sweet foods such as chocolate?

1 often

2 sometimes

3 never

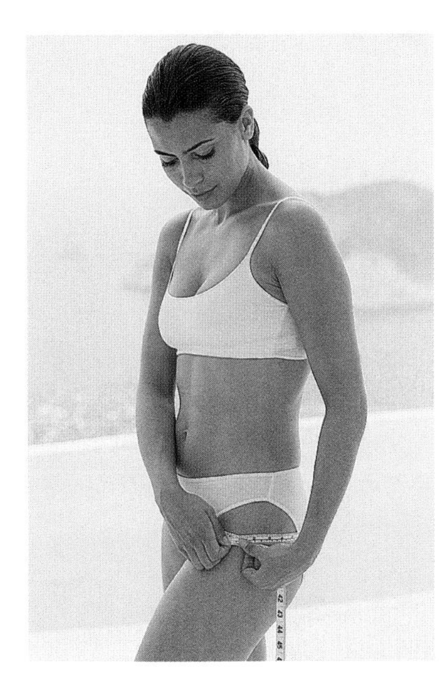

hip-to-waist ratio △

This test assesses your body shape and fat distribution. Measure your hips, then measure your waist (you can use either metric or imperial). Divide your waist measurement by your hip measurement.

1 **women: above 0.86**
  men: above 0.95
2 **women: 0.71–0.85**
  men: 0.81–0.94
3 **women: below 0.7**
  men: below 0.8

the one-minute crunch test ▽

The one-minute crunch test assesses your strength, and the postural strength of your tummy muscles, in particular. Perform as many crunches (*p21*) as you can in one minute. It doesn't matter too much if you have to stop and start, but make sure you keep your technique strong. Then compare the number you were able to do with the following scoring chart.

1 **women: 24 or below**
  men: 24 or below
2 **women: 25–45**
  men: 25–45
3 **women: 46 or more**
  men: 46 or more

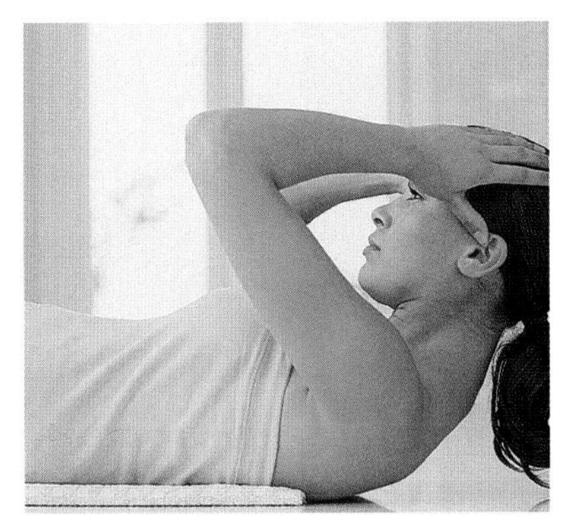

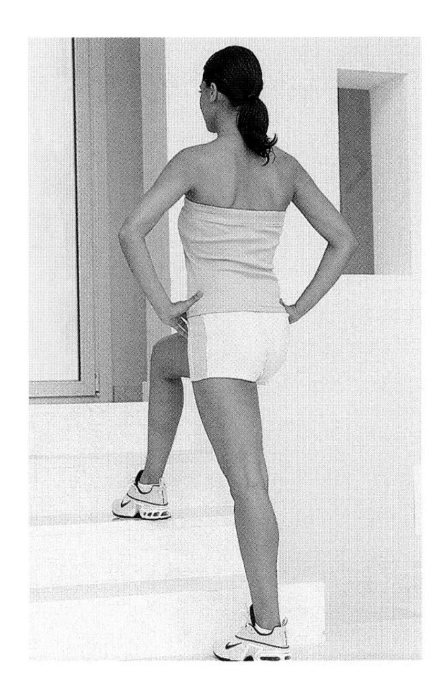

the step test △

This tests your cardiovascular fitness. Use a step or chair 16 in (40 cm) high and do step-ups (*p62*) at a rate of 30 per minute for 3 minutes. Stop, then take your pulse (*p17*) for 15 seconds. Multiply this figure by 4.

1 **women: 167 or more**
  men: 157 or more
2 **women: 141–166**
  men: 131–156
3 **women: 140 and below**
  men: 130 and below

---

working out your score

Add up your scores to the questions using the following scoring system:
1 = 1 point
2 = 2 points
3 = 3 points

Your total score decides your fitness level – either ① or ② – for the resistance work.

If you scored fewer than 35 points, you're fitness level ① – the easier of the two levels. If you scored 35 points or more, you're fitness level ② – the tougher level.

Don't worry if you're puzzled by why I'm asking some of the questions. I go into more detail about many of them later in the plan.

fat-burning cardio

Cardio training is what really burns fat. So, although it doesn't work in isolation, it is the most important part of the plan's workouts.

Cardio training – or aerobic exercise, as it's sometimes called – includes any activity that gets you out of breath. So running and fast-pace walking, cycling, and swimming all qualify as types of cardio work. Cardio training makes your heart and lungs work harder, and this does more than improve your physical fitness. It boosts your energy levels, improves your concentration, and reduces your risk of heart disease, too. Most importantly for those aiming to lose weight, cardio burns fat.

As you go about your day-to-day business, your body is drawing on its most readily available sources of energy – these are its fat reserves and the reserves of sugar held in your blood and muscles. At times like this, it uses them in roughly equal proportions. However, as soon as you ask your body to work harder, it needs the most immediate form of energy it has, and this it takes in the form of sugar. Although your body's now using proportionately more sugar than fat to fuel itself, it's still burning fat, and more fat than if you were simply going about your usual tasks.

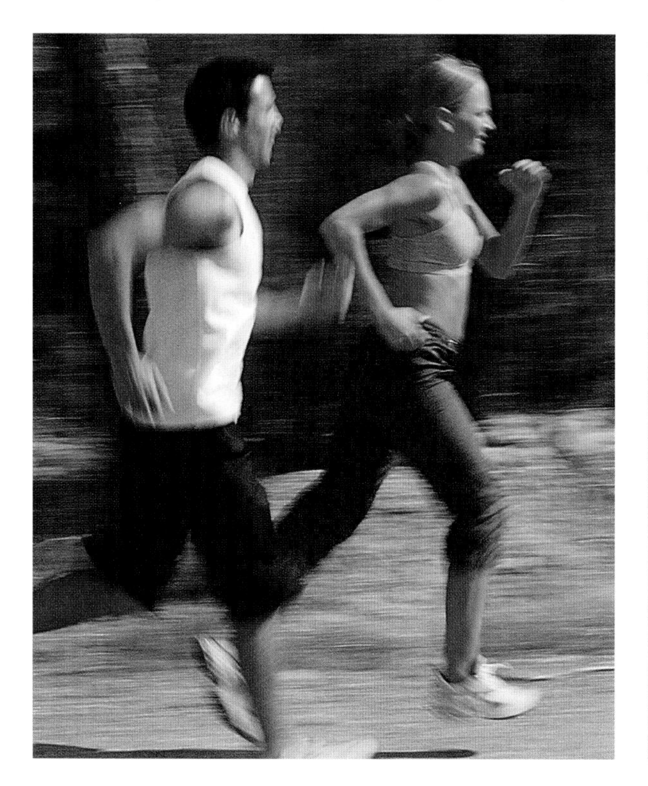

◁ To get your body working aerobically, running and fast-pace walking are part of the fat loss plan workouts.

▽ Swimming is an excellent form of cardio training. From day 23, you can incorporate it into your workouts.

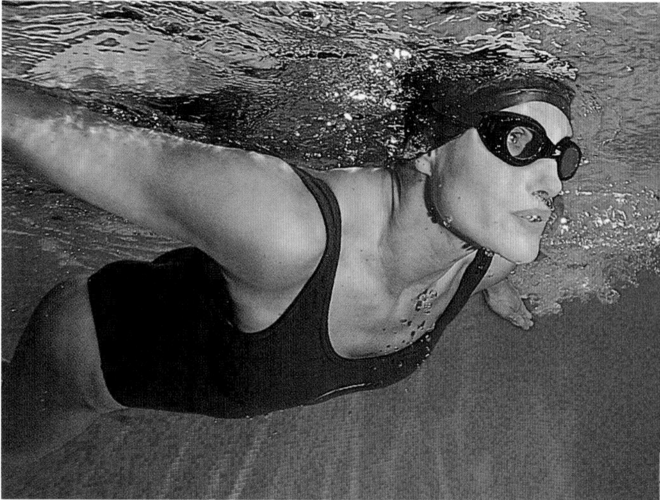

effective fat-burning

In the workouts, I'll ask you to perform cardio work in two different ways. The first, constant-pace training, has you working at a steady pace over a longer period – on day 1, for instance, you'll be walking at a constant pace for 25 minutes.

Interval training is the second way. Here, you'll alternate in the same session between short periods of low-intensity cardio training (walking) and short periods of high-intensity cardio training (running). You'll do this for the first time at the beginning of week two, when I ask you to fast-pace walk for a minute, then run for a minute.

This combination of constant-pace training and interval training makes your body burn fat in the most effective way it can. And the reason it works is that it raises your basal metabolic rate (BMR), which is the rate at which your body is calculated to burn calories when it's at rest.

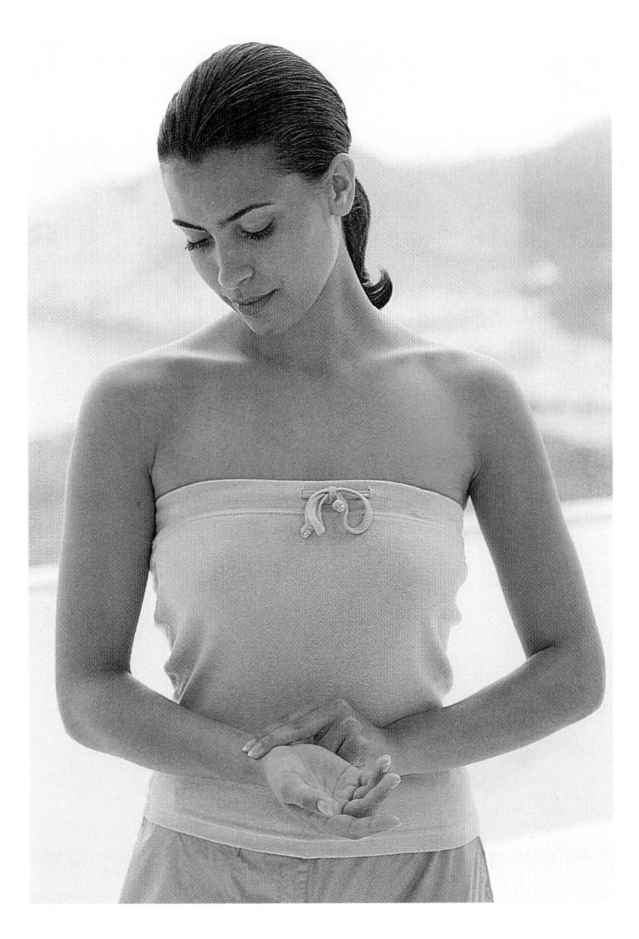

△ You need to take your pulse to know when you're working in your optimum training zone and burning fat most efficiently. The pulse at your wrist is probably the easiest to take. Check below for how to do it.

your optimum training zone

To burn fat efficiently, you also need to work within your optimum training zone, which is between 70% and 90% of your maximum heart rate (MHR).

Calculating your MHR may seem like a bit of bore to begin with, but you'll soon find you can recognize what heart rate you're working at by the way you feel, and there'll be no need for you to keep stopping and measuring it.

To work out your 100% MHR, assume that when you were born it was 220 and that it's going down by one each year. So, a 35-year-old has an MHR of 185 (220 – 35). With a calculator, you can then work out the MHR percentage you need. For example, the 80% MHR for a 35-year-old is 148 (0.8 x 185). This figure represents the maximum number of heartbeats per minute a 35-year-old should have during cardio work at 80% MHR. Don't worry if this seems complicated now. I'll run through it all again once you've begun the plan, and on page 156 there's a table of approximate figures to guide you.

The only other thing you need to know is how to take your pulse. Find the pulse point at your wrist by following the line of your thumb and placing two fingers (not your thumb) about 1 in (2 cm) below your wrist joint. Count for 15 seconds, then multiply by 4 to get your heartbeats per minute figure.

muscle-toning resistance

Resistance work is one of those terms you may hear bandied around, but what does it actually mean? And how will it help you reshape your body?

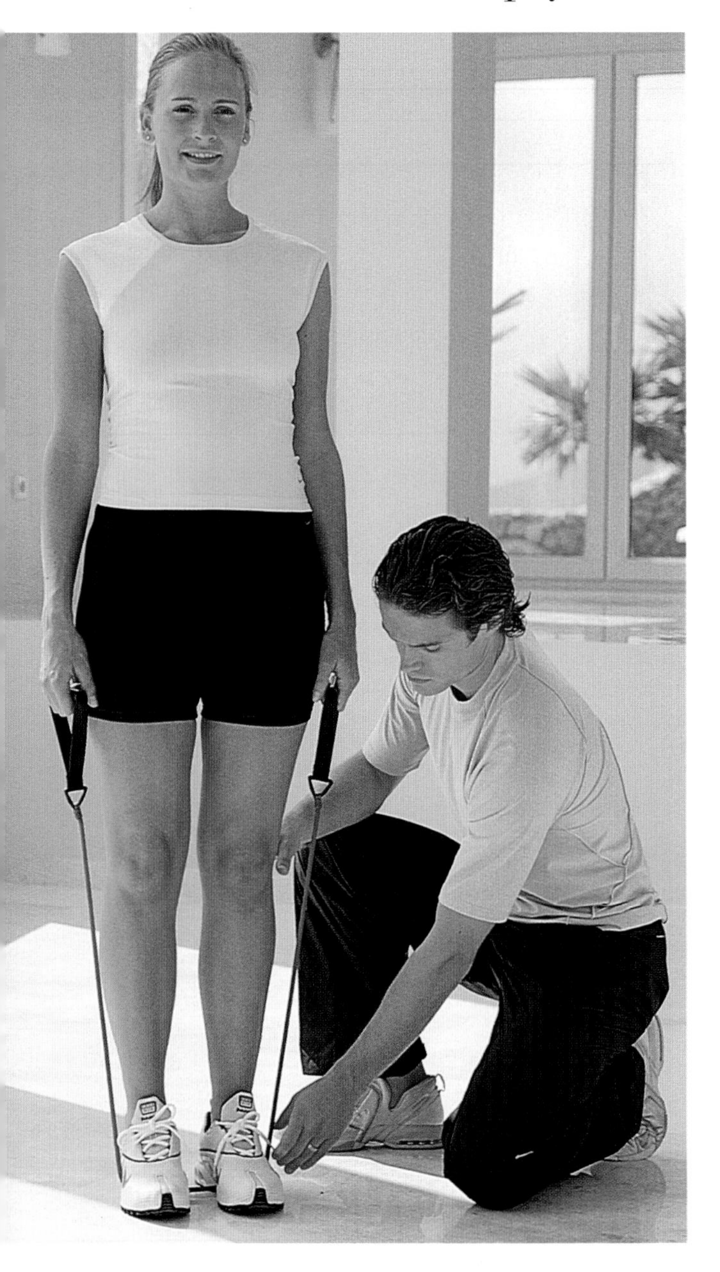

If the term sounds unfamiliar to you, the activities it describes won't. Toning, pumping, body pump, matrix, sculpting – these are all forms of resistance work. The reason they're known as resistance work is that they all work one particular muscle – or one particular group of muscles – with the help of some kind of resistance, whether that's an exertube, hand weight, or simply your own body weight. So when you're toning your tummy muscles with a crunch, or sculpting your upper arms with a bicep curl and exertube, you're performing resistance work. And resistance work is crucial in the process of losing body fat and improving your shape.

why is it so special?

Your muscles are the energy-burning part of your body – the better the condition they're in, the greater your body's ability to burn calories. Resistance training works your muscles hard, and, by forcing them to adapt to new 'loads,' you're making them – and your body – more efficient.

does it make you bulky?

This is a question I'm often asked, and the answer is 'no.' Creating 'body mass' is actually very hard.

◁ Exercising with an exertube is an integral part of my fat loss plan workouts. If you've never used one before, take the time to get the hang of it. Two of the startup exercises on page 21 call for this simple piece of equipment.

To achieve it, bodybuilders and others have to work in a specific way. And this is not it.

The aim of my resistance programs is to make every single fiber of your body perform to its absolute potential. By varying the speed at which you exercise, the number of 'reps' you perform (*see below*), and the order you perform them in, I've made sure you're never at any risk of producing continuous growth in one area. If you find your jeans don't fit in quite the way you want them to after exercising, don't worry – you're not bulking up. Your body is recovering from its exertions. Everything will be back to normal in a few hours.

what are reps?

When you come to the resistance programs, you'll see that for every exercise, I give you a number of 'reps' to perform according to your fitness level. A rep (repetition) is one complete performance of an exercise from start to finish. So, when I ask you for 10 reps, you perform that particular exercise a total of 10 times. The precise time a rep should take varies from exercise to exercise, but as a rough rule of thumb, allow

- 4 secs per rep if you're doing 10–12 reps
- 3 secs per rep if you're doing 15–18 reps
- 2 secs per rep if you're doing 20+ reps

the resistance startup

To get you used to resistance work, I've put together a startup session of five exercises (*p20–21*). Practice these until you feel absolutely confident about what you're doing. Two of them require an exertube, so you'll also be getting the hang of using that. Once you're started the fat loss plan and the days begin to tick by, I'll introduce you to more resistance exercises, so that by the end of the eight weeks you'll have a repertoire of 40.

▽ Resistance work doesn't always require a resistance prop. Your own body weight will do, as in this exercise, the back extension (*p38*). Resistance exercises using your own body weight are another vital part of the workouts.

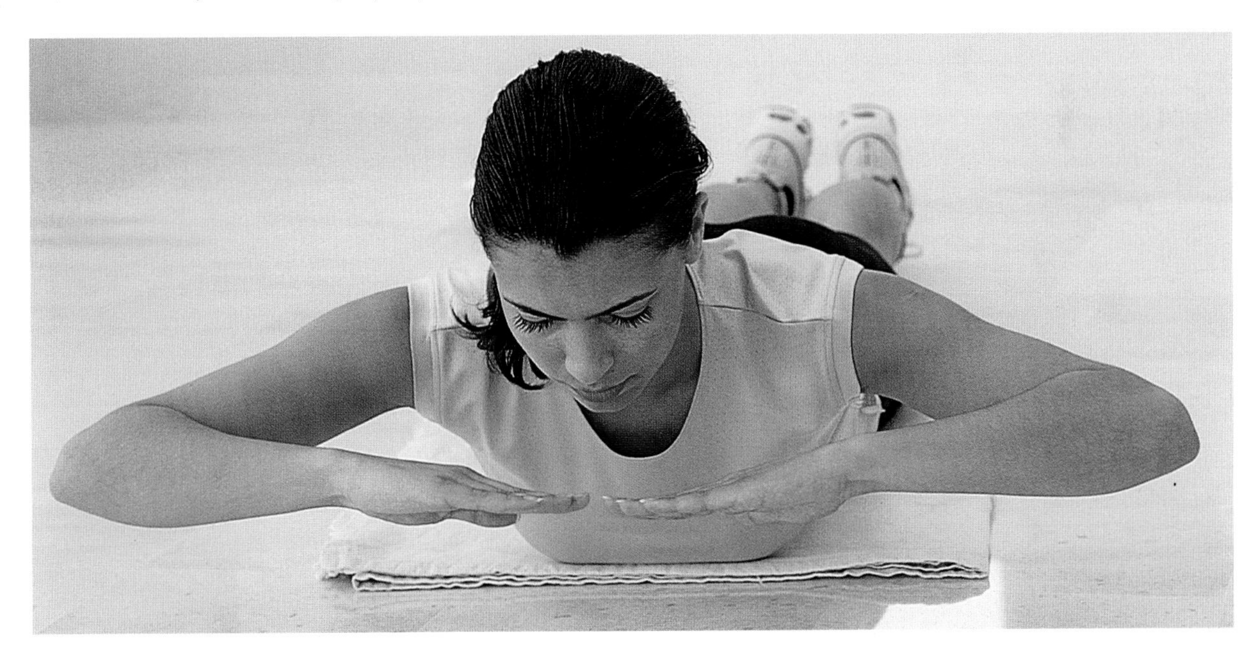

resistance startup

To get you in the swing of things for your first big day, here are five resistance exercises that will start the work on the major muscle groups of your body.

Before you start day 1 of the plan, I recommend you take some time to practice the kind of resistance exercises you'll be doing, and get used to using your exertube. Study these step-by-steps, then repeat the exercises until your body is stable, safe, and working hard. Once you're confident it is, you're ready to pick your day to start losing fat.

squat ▷

Squats are the classic exercise for working your thighs and buttocks, as well as the muscles of your lower leg and lower back. These burn more calories than any other muscles.

1 Stand with your feet hip-width apart, knees slightly bent. Put your hands on your hips and keep your back straight.

2 Bend your knees to 90° and lean your body forward until it's at a right angle to your thighs. Keep your heels on the floor. Slowly raise yourself to the start position.

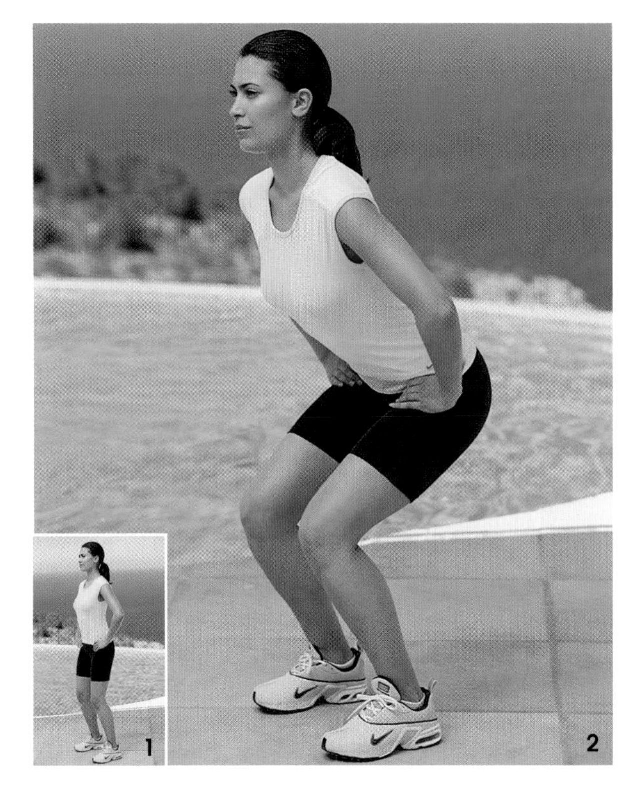

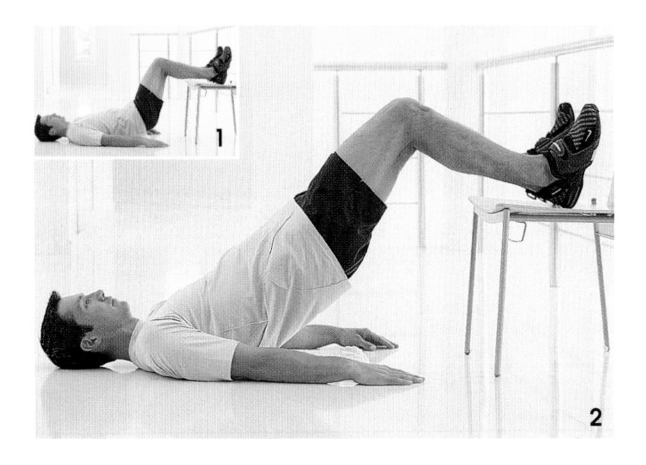

body raise ◁

Intensive work for your butt and the backs of your legs. If pointing your toes away from you in Step 2 is too tricky, leave them pointing directly up.

1 Lie on your back with your heels on a chair and your knees at 90°. Place your arms by your sides, palms down.

2 Raise your pelvis until your body is straight from your knees to your chest. Pointing your toes away from you, squeeze your buttocks. Don't allow your chest to bow. Slowly lower yourself to the start position.

bicep curl ▷

For lean-looking arms, you need to tone your biceps. The bicep curl does the job to perfection.

1 Hold the exertube with a handle in each hand and place your feet hip-width apart in the middle of it, knees slightly bent. Start with your arms by your sides and your elbows slightly bent. Your palms should face forward.

2 Bend your arms and lift the handles up toward your shoulders. Keep your back straight and your elbows tucked in close to your body. When your arms are at shoulder height, flex your biceps to maximize the effectiveness of the exercise. Slowly lower your arms to the start position.

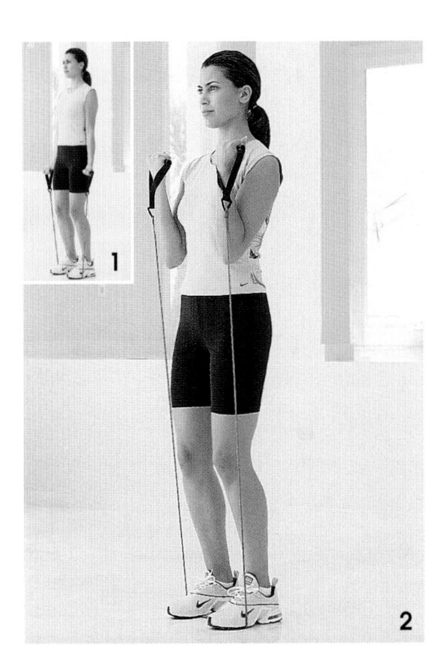

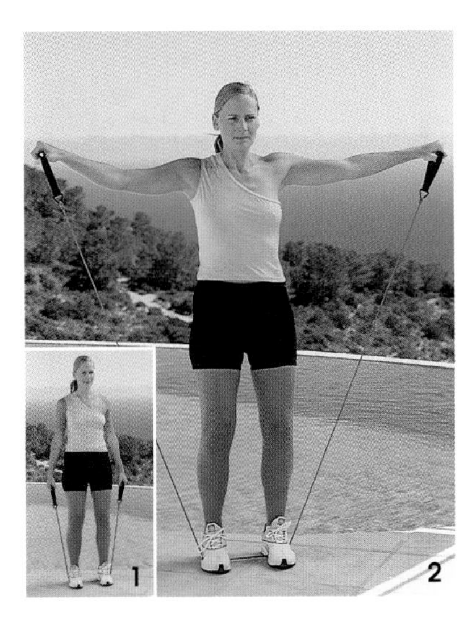

lateral raise ◁

The lateral raise tones your biceps and triceps for those desirable V-shaped arms.

1 Hold the exertube with a handle in each hand and place your feet hip-width apart in the middle of it, knees slightly bent. Start with your arms by your sides, palms facing inward. Keep your back straight and your tummy muscles pulled in.

2 Keeping your elbows slightly bent, slowly raise your arms away from your sides until your hands are level with your shoulders. Keep your palms facing down toward the floor and your torso as still as possible. Slowly lower your arms to the start position.

crunch ▷

This is one of the most basic stomach exercises, but it's also highly effective and very easy to do.

1 Lie on your back with your knees bent and your feet flat on the floor. Place your hands by your ears.

2 Breathe out, curling your shoulders forward as you do so. Keep your lower back on the floor and your tummy muscles pulled in. Maintain a space the size of your fist under your chin so your head stays in line with your spine. Return to the start position, breathing in as you do so.

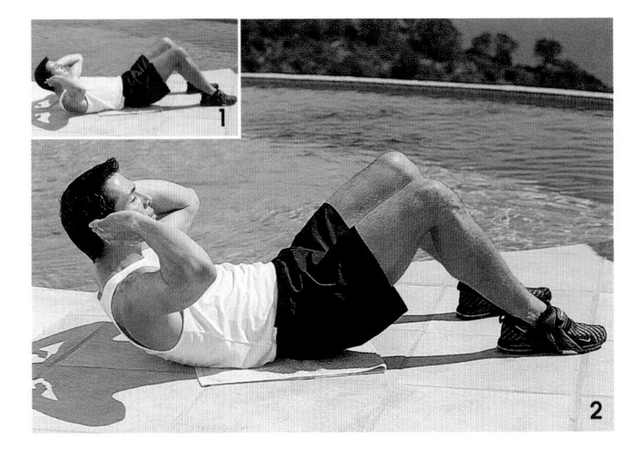

cooling-down stretches

In much the same way as you warm your muscles up before resistance exercise, so you have to cool them down afterward with flexibility-enhancing stretches.

Strange as it may sound, exercise actually reduces your flexibility – by making your muscles shorten and contract. That's why it's essential to stretch immediately after exercising, when your muscles are warmed up and at their most responsive. With the right stretches, you can head off stiffness, reduce the risk of injury, and create good flexibility.

I've chosen three stretch sequences for you. Which one I ask you to do at the end of each workout depends on the kind of exercise you've been doing. Generally, it will be a lower body stretch or total body stretch (although you can substitute a short standing stretch for this if time is short). I explain each move in full on pages 24–27.

total body stretch takes 5–10 minutes

Although it takes a little longer than the other two, this stretch is worth it. It will leave you feeling like a new person. Keep your breathing slow and controlled throughout.

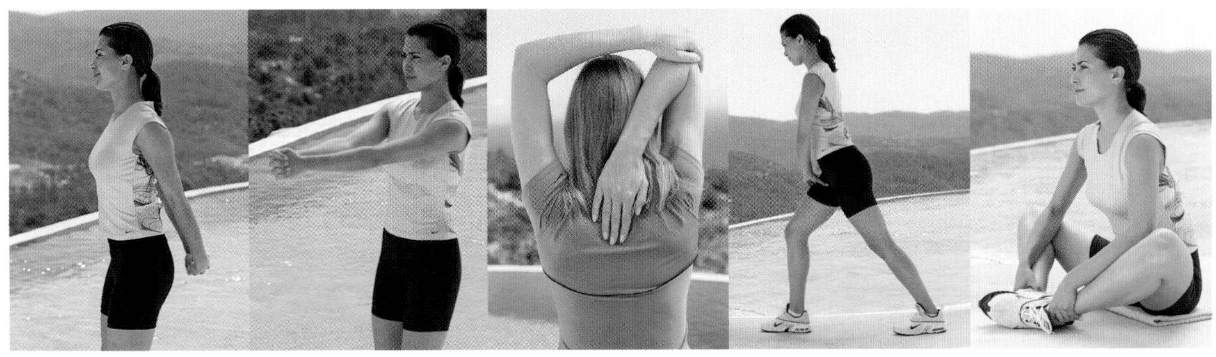

chest stretch *p24* hold for 15 sec | upper back stretch *p24* hold for 15 sec | tricep stretch *p24* hold for 10 sec | calf stretch *p27* hold for 20 sec | inner thigh stretch *p27* hold for 30+ sec

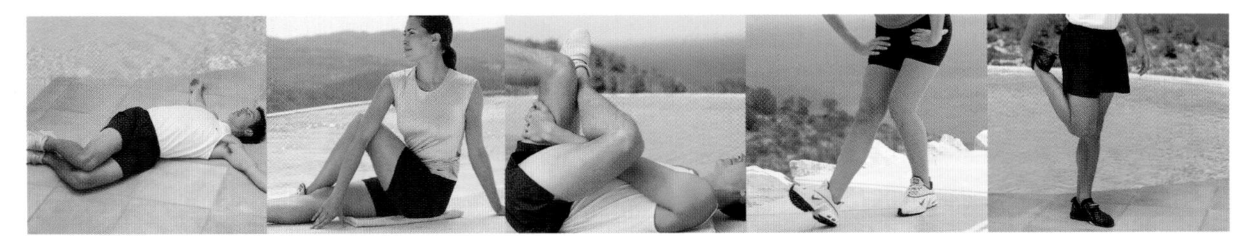

spine rotation *p25* hold for 15 sec | outer thigh stretch *p27* hold for 30+ sec | glute stretch *p25* hold for 15+ sec | hamstring stretch *p26* hold for 20 sec | quadricep stretch *p26* hold for 20 sec

lower body stretch takes 5 minutes

When you have the time after an intense lower body toning resistance program, or after a run or fast-pace walk, this sequence will give you the ultimate lower body stretch.

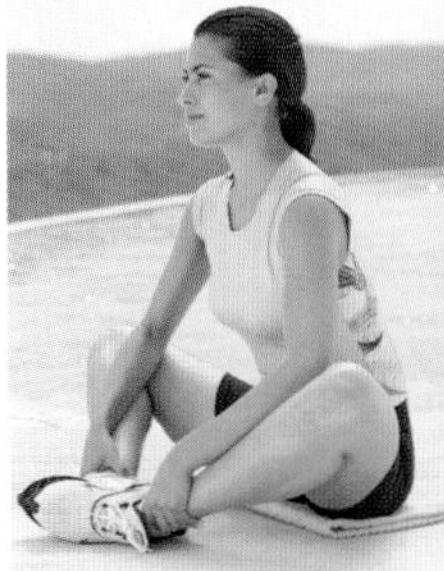

inner thigh stretch *p27*
hold for 30+ sec

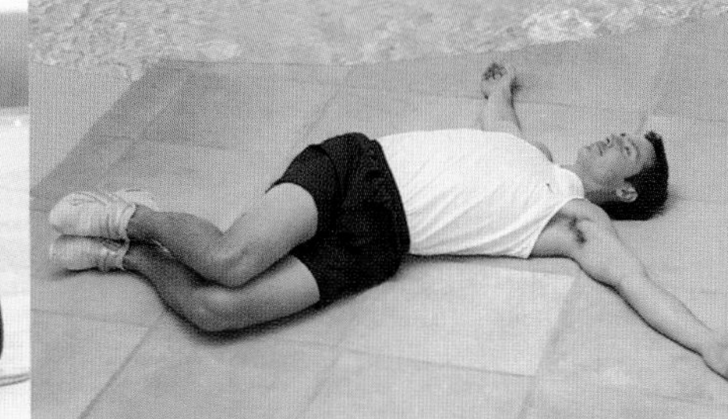

spine rotation *p25*
hold for 15 sec

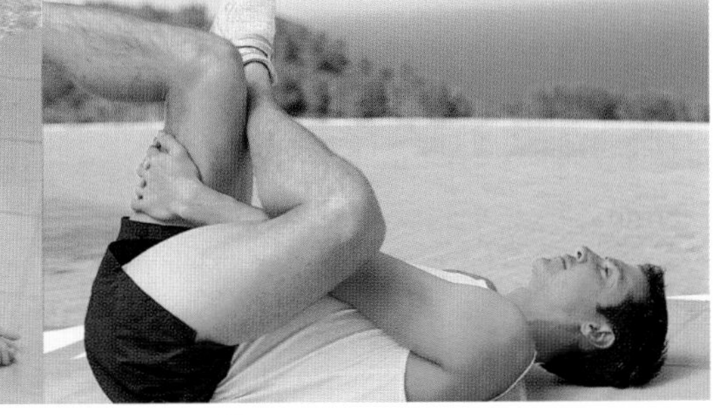

glute stretch *p25*
hold for 15+ sec

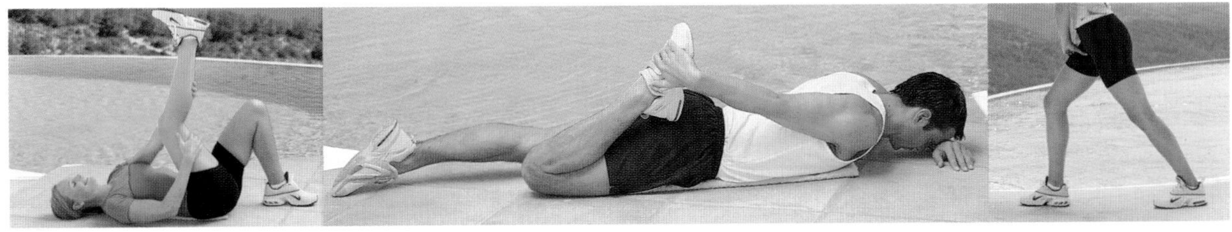

hamstring stretch *p25*
hold for 30 sec

quadricep stretch (lying down) *p26*
hold for 20 sec

calf stretch *p27*
hold for 20 sec

short standing stretch takes 5 minutes

Ideal for cooling down after a run or fast-pace walk, or for those occasions when you're pressed for time, the short standing stretch features a few quick exercises for all the major muscle groups.

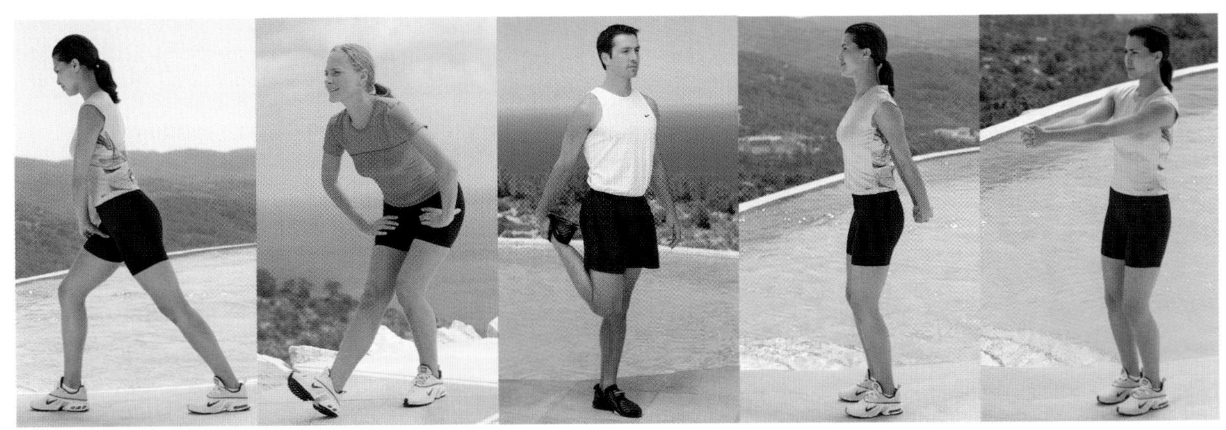

calf stretch *p27*
hold for 20 sec

hamstring stretch *p26*
hold for 20 sec

quadricep stretch *p26*
hold for 20 sec

chest stretch *p24*
hold for 15 sec

upper back stretch *p24*
hold for 15 sec

the stretch moves

By stretching the muscles in your arms, chest, back, and legs, you're eliminating tension, building good flexibility, and reducing soreness. Although I've put these stretch moves in sequences for you to perform at the end of each workout, you can also perform each stretch on its own at other times. This is useful if one particular area of your body is feeling stiff and sore. If you feel a little wobbly when you do the standing hamstring and quadricep stretches, hold on to a wall or rail.

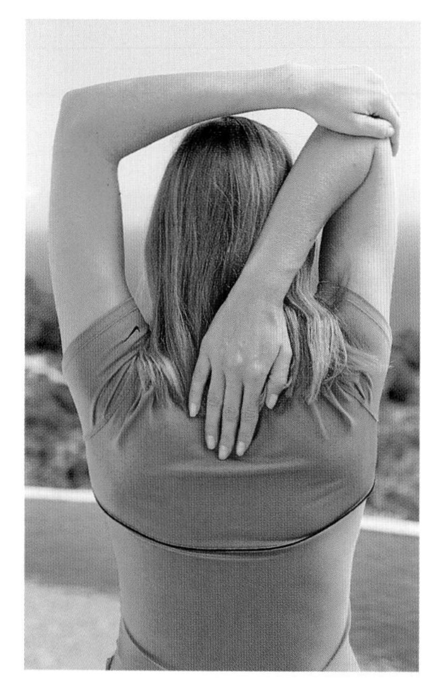

tricep stretch △

Stand with your feet hip-width apart and your legs slightly bent. Raise one arm and place the hand over your back (as if you were reaching down your spine). Now increase the stretch by gently pushing the elbow back with your other hand. Hold the position, feeling the stretch down the back of your arm, for 10 seconds. Slowly return to the start position and repeat with the other arm.

chest stretch ▽

Stand with your feet hip-width apart and your legs slightly bent. Pull your tummy muscles in and keep your head, neck, and shoulders relaxed. Clasp your hands behind your back. Keeping your back straight, lift your arms behind you until you can feel the stretch across your chest. Hold for 15 seconds, then return to the start.

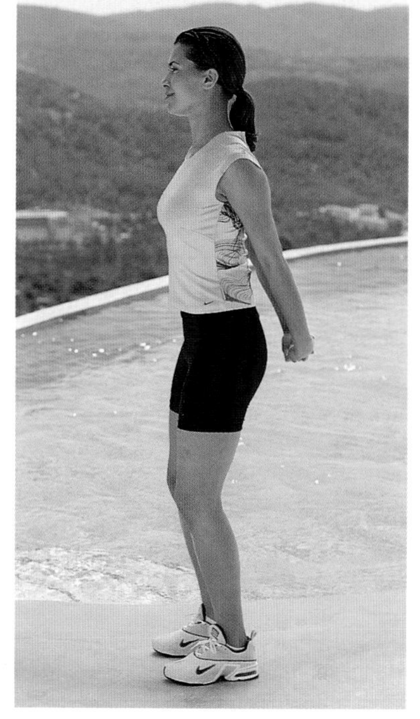

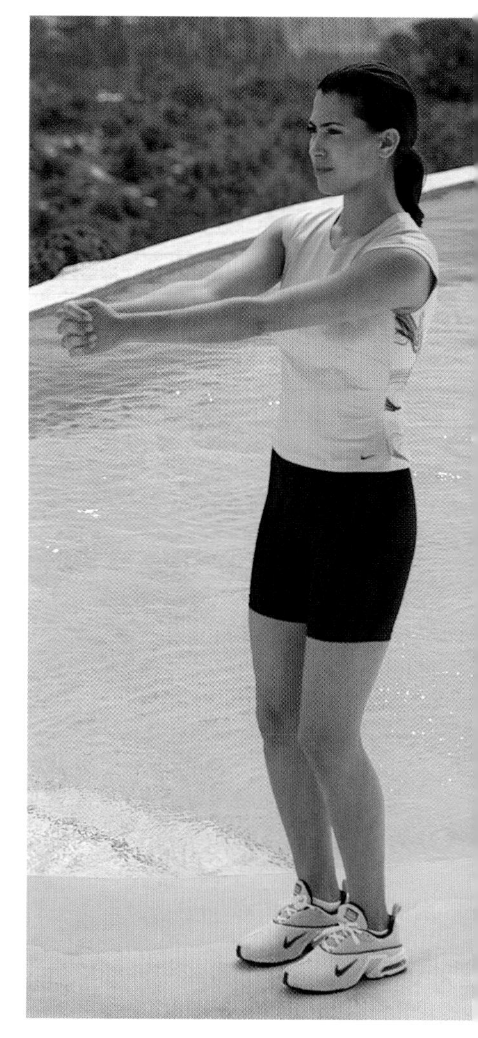

upper back stretch △

Stand with your feet hip-width apart and your legs slightly bent. Straighten your arms out in front of you and clasp your fingers together. Keeping your lower back firm and your body upright, gently push your hands away from you. Feel the stretch across your upper back and at the back of your shoulders. Hold for about 15 seconds and then slowly lower your arms to the start position.

spine rotation ▷

Lie on your back, with arms stretched out at shoulder level. Bend both legs to 90°, then drop your knees to one side so one is touching the floor. Keep your shoulder blades flat on the floor, but don't force the stretch. Hold for 15 seconds, then return to the start before repeating on the other side.

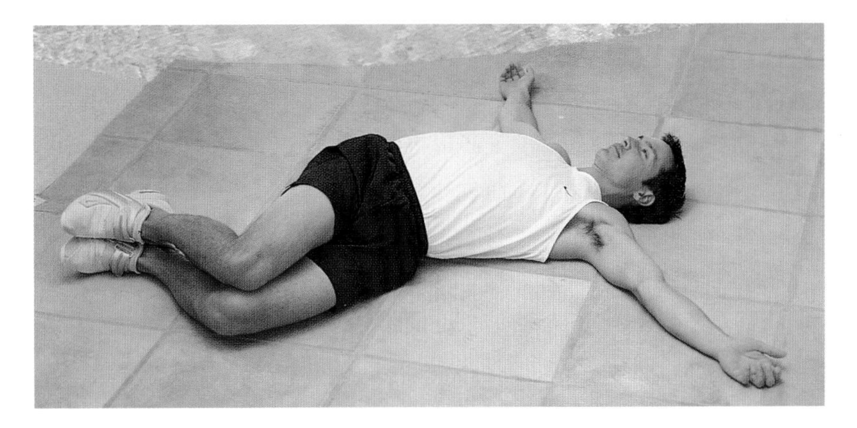

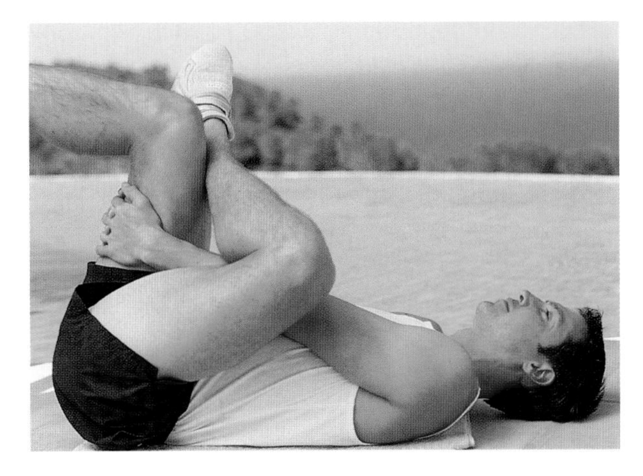

glute stretch ◁

Lie on your back on the floor. Bend the knee of one leg, but keep your foot on the floor. Cross your other leg over your first leg so your ankle is resting just above the knee. Clasp the thigh of your first leg firmly by both hands, then gently pull it toward you. Feel the stretch in your bottom and your outer thigh. Hold the position for about 15 seconds (or a little longer if you can), then slowly return your legs to the start position. Repeat the stretch using your other leg.

hamstring stretch ▷ (lying down)

Lie on your back on the floor with one leg bent at the knee and your foot flat on the floor. Hold your other leg with one hand behind the thigh and one hand behind the calf. Keeping this leg as straight as you can, gently pull it toward you until you feel the stretch down the back of your thigh. Hold the position for 30 seconds, allowing the muscle to relax into the stretch as you do so. Slowly return to the start position. Repeat with the other leg.

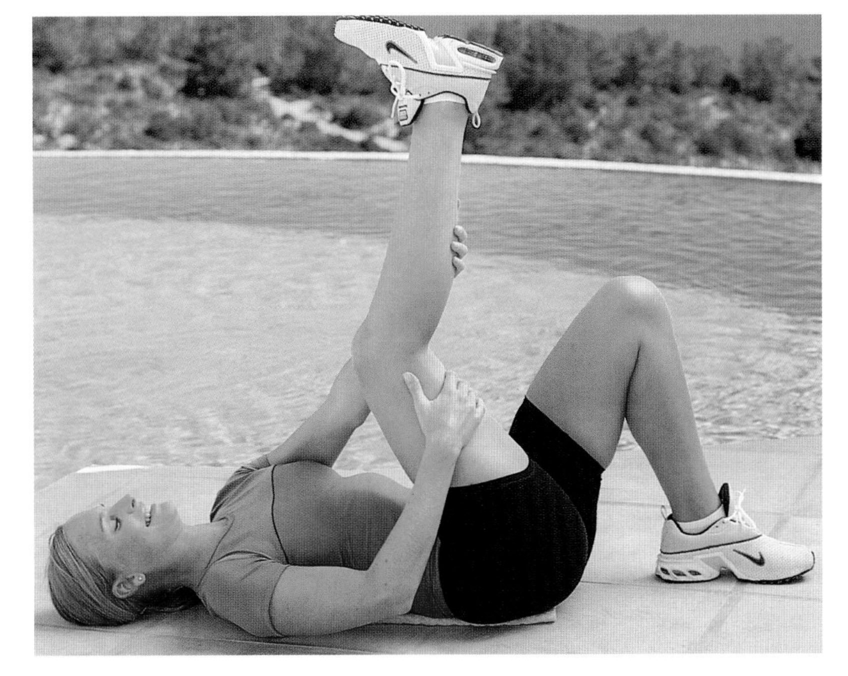

hamstring stretch ▷

Place one heel in front of you and put your hands on your thighs. Bend your other knee and slowly bend forward from the hips. Feel the stretch in the back of your thigh, calf, and the back of your knee. Hold for 10 seconds, then slowly lean in a little farther to intensify the stretch. Hold for 10 seconds, then repeat on the other side.

quadricep stretch ▽

Stand up straight, keeping your supporting leg slightly bent. Bend your other leg and, holding the front of your foot, pull it up toward your bottom. Keep your knees together, hips pointing forward, and back straight. Feel the stretch in the front of your thigh and your hip. Hold for 20 seconds, then repeat with the other leg.

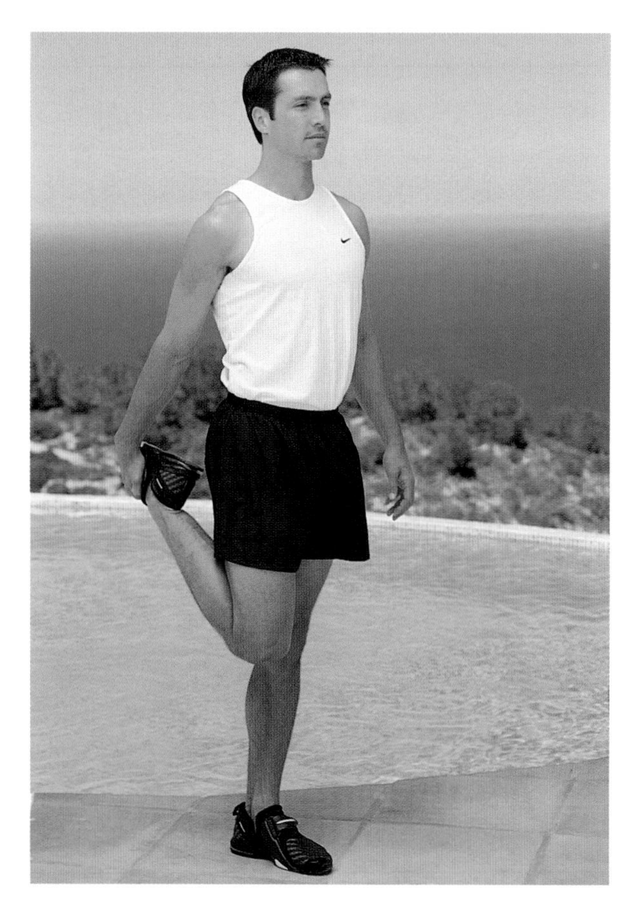

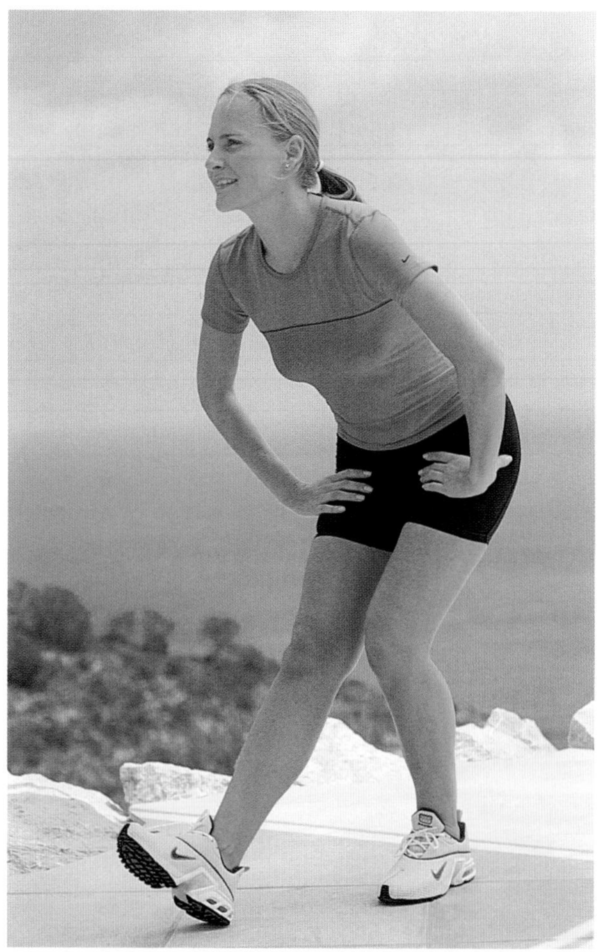

quadricep stretch (lying down) ▽

Lie face down with your head on one hand. Keeping your hips on the floor, bring one leg behind you and hold the front of the foot. Keep your head down and neck relaxed. Hold for 20 seconds, then repeat with the other leg.

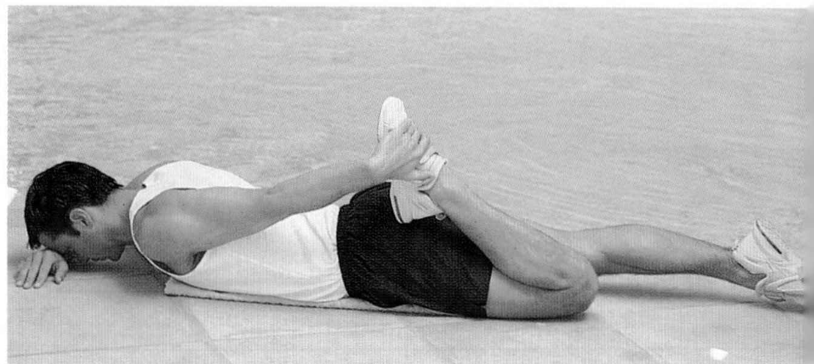

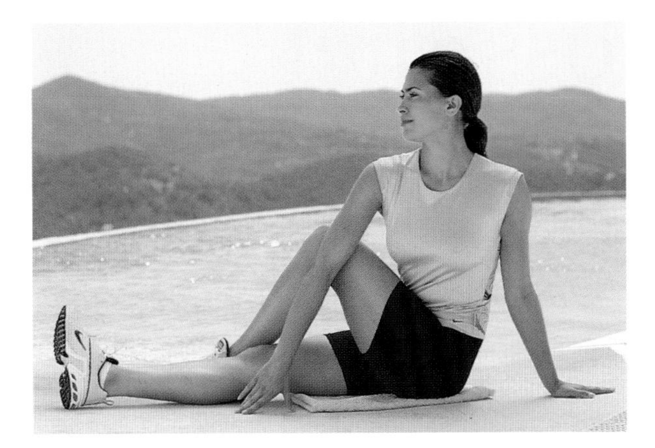

outer thigh stretch △

Sit with one leg out in front of you and the other crossed over it. With one arm for support, use the other to ease your knee across your body. Feel the stretch in your outer thigh. Hold for 30 seconds. Repeat with your other leg.

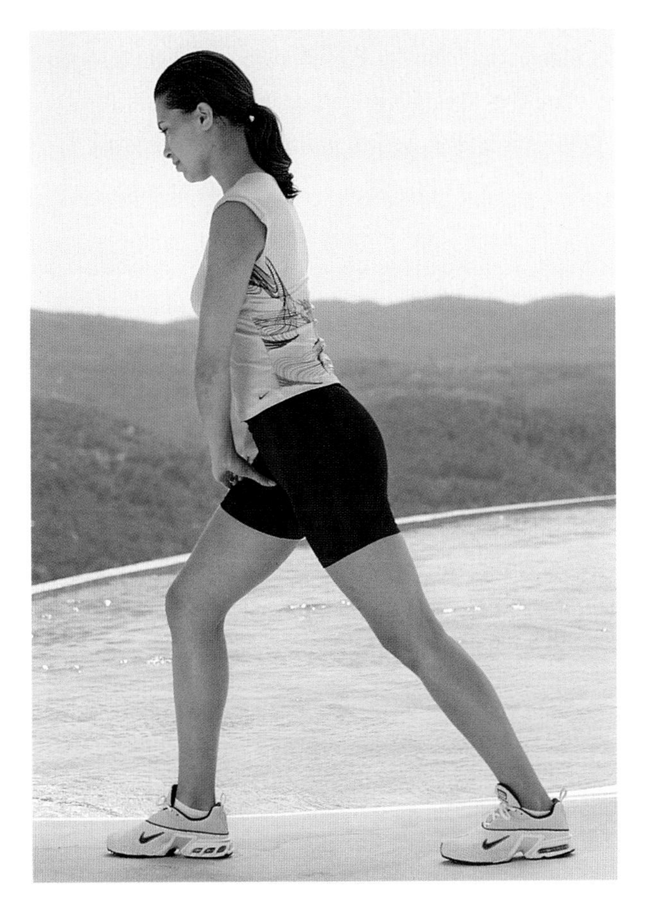

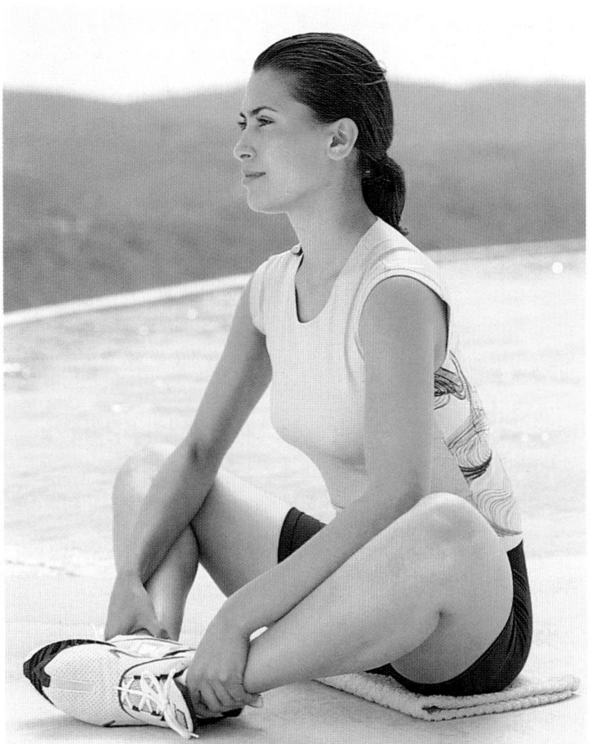

inner thigh stretch △

Sit with your back straight. Place the soles of your feet together, then, holding your ankles, pull your feet in toward you. Hold the stretch for 30 seconds, feeling it in your inner thighs as you relax your legs down toward the floor. You can intensify this stretch by placing your elbows on your knees and, keeping your back straight, gently easing your body forward from the hips.

calf stretch ◁

Stand with feet together, then step back with one foot, pushing into the heel and bending your other leg slightly. Keep your back straight, feet facing forward, and heels on the floor. Imagine a straight line running from your back heel to your head. Hold for about 20 seconds, feeling the stretch in your calf. Repeat with your other leg. You can intensify this stretch by moving your rear foot slightly back, pushing into the heel, and holding for a few seconds.

a healthy fat loss diet

A varied diet of good, tasty food is essential for achieving fat loss. Far from being dull and virtuous, it's a delicious recipe for success – as you'll soon agree.

Whenever I start talking about a healthy diet, I can almost see the thoughts running through people's heads. 'The food is going to be boring.' 'I'll have to use strange, healthy ingredients.' 'The food will have no taste.' And what strikes me immediately is that these people have put up a kind of barrier: they simply don't realize that healthy eating isn't a question of turning your life upside-down. Switching to a healthy diet is all about changing your attitude toward food, experimenting, and having fun.

Our daily enjoyment of the food we eat is an important psychological relaxant. The perfect diet should let us savor food without ever leaving us feeling guilty (there are always going to be times we end up indulging, after all). It should also be good for us, and the best way to work out if a diet's healthy or not is to apply the 80/20 rule. According to this 80/20 rule, around 80% of the food you eat should be healthy – the kind I feature in the fat loss plan. The other 20% of the time, you're free to enjoy the foods you really like – even if they don't always feature on my list of healthy foods (*p30–31*). You just can't go crazy.

For me, food should be a **joyful** experience and not the enemy. The **perfect diet** should let us savor food without ever leaving us feeling guilty.

my fat loss diet

The diet I'm asking you to follow over the next eight weeks is not quite 80/20. That's because I've designed the fat loss plan to help you lose fat quickly. The foods I've chosen are 100% healthy, 100% of the time. When you've completed the plan, you can reintroduce your favorite treats (*see* 'eating to stay lean' *on pages 154–156*).

Variety is one important factor I had in mind as I planned the recipes at the back of the book. Our bodies respond favorably to being given different types of food and digesting different nutrients from different sources.

'Eating with the seasons' is something else I consider important. This was the way our ancestors ate, and they had a diet that varied throughout the year. The chances are that seasonal food is fresher, too, so you get the most of its goodness.

Speaking of goodness, many of the ingredients you'll be eating are raw, since this is by far the best way to eat them. When you do cook them, you'll use methods like steaming, grilling, roasting, and stir-frying, which keep the goodness in.

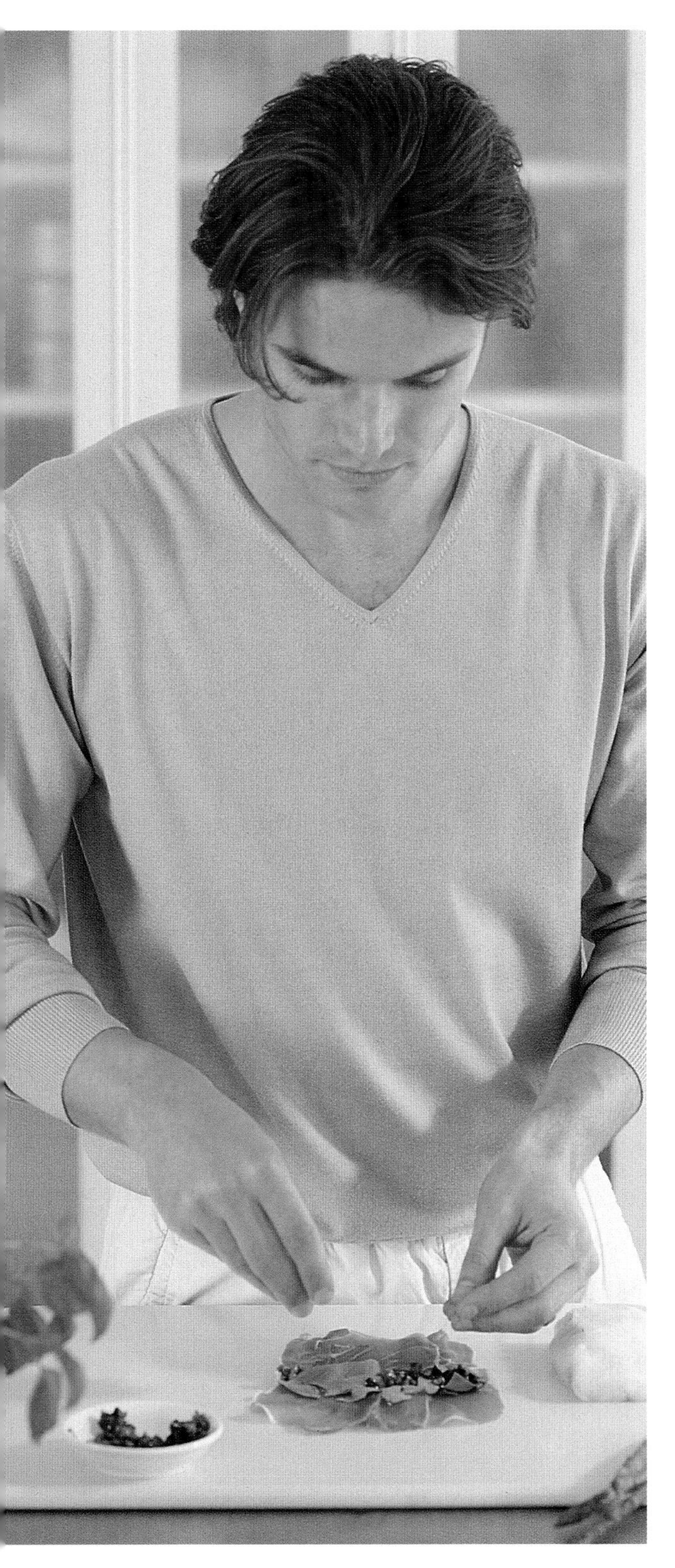

protein, carbs, and fat

In the fat loss plan recipes, I've kept a close eye on the quantities of proteins, fat, and carbs (carbohydrates). These are the main food groups of our daily diet, and our bodies need all of them – in the right proportions – to keep us healthy.

Each day for the next eight weeks, you have the choice between two breakfast dishes, two lunch dishes, and two dinners. Whichever you choose, you'll get a healthy balance of protein, carbs, and fat. I've even included a scoring system, so you can see which kinds of food are high in protein, say, and which are low in fat.

snacks and calories

I'm in favor of strategic snacking. A midmorning and midafternoon snack are essential, in fact, to ward off energy lows. Each day, I've given you a selection of foods to snack on – it's up to you what you have when. Men are allowed more snacks than women because they have a higher metabolic rate and consume more calories.

The calorie count I've allowed you each day is 1,700 cal if you're a woman, and 1,900 cal if you're a man. This is about 500 cal per day fewer than your body will be expending. In combination with the workouts, you're all set to lose fat.

a note about alcohol

Throughout the course of the plan, I want you to avoid alcohol. I know it sounds tough, but if you really want to change, let's do it right.

◁ Monkfish wrapped in Parma ham (*p146*) may be among the most luxurious dishes you'll have while you're on the fat loss plan, but it's still very, very healthy.

foods to eat more...
...and foods to eat less

Eating a diet of fresh, healthy foods sounds simple. But there's more to it than that: while some foods are clearly ideal, others are much less obvious bad guys.

One useful way of classifying food is by the glycemic index. This lists foods by how quickly they affect the body's blood-sugar levels. According to the index, fruit and legumes are low-glycemic. That's because they're sources of slow-release energy that don't cause the energy peaks and troughs that make you want to snack.

The staples of many western diets, on the other hand, like potatoes, cereals, and sugary foods, are often high-glycemic. They're sources of quick-release energy that fuel the body rapidly with sugar – and just as quickly leave it craving more.

acid and alkaline

As much as possible, I eat foods that my body can break down easily, since I believe they clean up our systems for us. Alkaline foods, as I call them, fight against oxidation by neutralizing free radicals. At the same time, I avoid foods that are difficult to digest. They're acid-forming, and create more toxic by-products as our bodies break them down.

Here, I've grouped everyday foods according to their glycemic index rating and their acid/alkaline effect on the body. From this, you can tell at a glance which you should be eating more and which you should be eating less.

eat more

low-glycemic alkaline food. The following should make up 40% of your weekly diet

fruit

apples
avocados
berries
dates (fresh)
figs (fresh)
grapes
kiwis
limes
mangoes
melons (except cantaloupe and watermelons)
pineapple

vegetables

asparagus
broccoli
Brussels sprouts
cabbage
carrots
cauliflower
celery
chicory
cucumber
eggplant
ginger
kale
leeks
peppers
squash
sweet potatoes
spinach
turnips
zucchini

grains

Camargue red rice
millet
quinoa
rice noodles
semolina
wholegrain rice
wild rice

legumes

cannellini beans
lima beans
chickpeas
kidney beans
lentils
peas
soybeans

nuts and seeds

almonds
brazil nuts
chestnuts
sesame seeds

fish & poultry

chicken
firm white fish
oily fish
turkey

oils

olive oil
safflower oil
sesame oil

eat more

medium-glycemic alkaline food. The following should make up 30% of your diet

fruit

strawberries

grains & pasta

corn pasta
couscous
polenta
rice pasta
light rye bread
whole-wheat pasta

seeds

pumpkin seeds
sunflower seeds

dairy products & their alternatives

dairy-free milk like soy milk and rice milk
low-fat plain yogurt
skim milk

eat less

high-glycemic food. The following should make up less than 10% of your diet

sugars

honey
sugar
corn syrup & maple syrup

vegetables

potatoes
parsnips
rutabagas

grains

bagels
dark rye bread

fruit

bananas
dried fruit

eat less

acid-forming food. The following should make up less than 20% of your diet

dairy products

butter
cheese
cream
whole milk
whole-milk sweetened yogurt

grains & wheat

basmati rice
cookies & cake
croissants
pasta (excluding whole-wheat)
pastries
sweetened breakfast cereals
sweetened rice puffs
wheat flakes
white bread, including French bread

fruit

citrus fruit
cranberries
plums
prunes
tomatoes

nuts

cashews
peanuts

other

alcohol
chocolate
coffee
potato chips
processed foods
red meat
tea

your lifestyle, my diet

Forward planning is as important as diet for successful fat loss. Pinpoint potential trouble spots now, and later you'll resist anything – including temptation.

There are times in all our lives when we get home a little later than anticipated and we're hungry. Somehow or other we find ourselves heading straight for the refrigerator. For many of us this is a make-or-break situation: give in to temptation now and we can all too easily end up feeling demoralized and down. With some careful organization, however, you can tackle the problem head-on – and satisfy your hunger pangs.

plan your grocery shopping

The way I've arranged the fat loss plan, you can see at a glance the meals and snacks you'll be eating over the coming days. From that, it's a simple matter of planning your shopping trip around the food you need. Not only will your fridge be stocked with ingredients for meals that are quick and healthy, but your diet – and your confidence – will remain intact.

Quite a few of my recipes call for canned ingredients like tuna, beans, or olives. Beware of hidden calories when you're buying these: they may come in sugary water or oil, which can increase your calorie intake. Look for products packed in plain water, or without added sugar at least. Don't worry that you'll be losing out on flavor – I'll show you how to maximize that with herbs and spices.

The best spreads for sandwiches and toast, by the way, are the nonhydrogenated kinds. Unlike many old-fashioned margarines, these are soft. They're also low in cholesterol. Even so, use only a scraping. Look for them at the supermarket – they should be clearly labeled as containing no hydrogenated fats or oils.

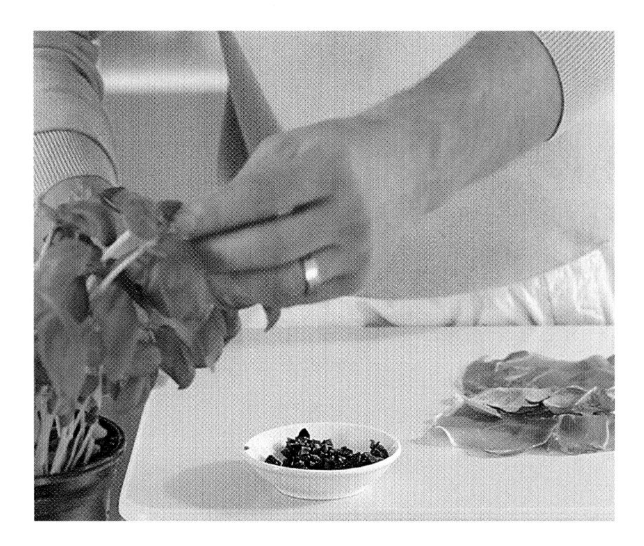

preparing ahead

Another aim of mine was to help you put together meals as quickly as possible. In the recipe section at the back of the book, I've indicated when some of the preparation or cooking can be done ahead of time. Most often, it's for dishes where ingredients

◁ Have fresh herbs to hand whenever possible. They'll add loads of flavor to your cooking, where commercially prepared foods rely on fats and sugars. The difference is not just in the flavor – it's in the calorie count, too.

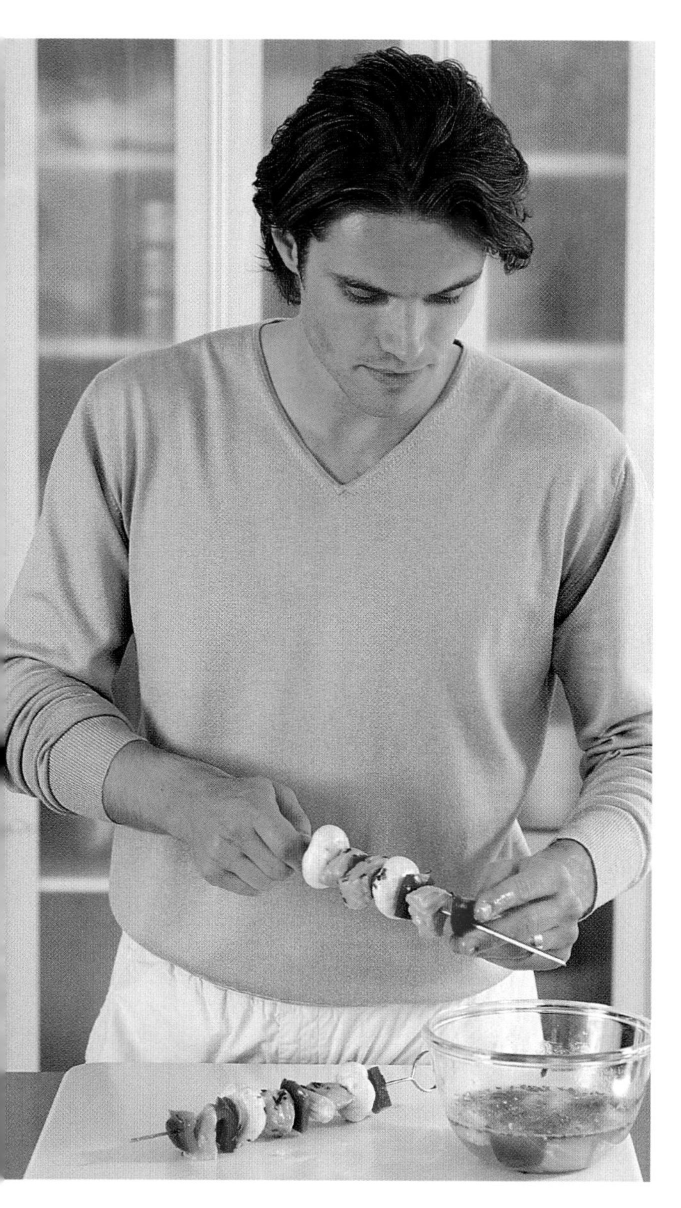

◁ As well as adding lots of flavor, marinating allows you to work up to 24 hours ahead, cutting down on the preparation time when you're ready to eat. The kabobs on pages 142–143 are ideal for this treatment.

need to be marinated. These can usually be left in the fridge for up to 24 hours. Many of the dressings, too, can be whizzed up beforehand. You could even get into the habit of making enough for several dishes at a time. They generally keep well.

strong, tasty flavors

As someone who loves good food, eating for the sake of eating is not my philosophy. The variety of flavors and textures of food are too important to me for that. Satisfying your taste buds with delicious food is also an excellent way of stopping your eyes from roaming around for more once you've eaten. The flavor does have to be there in the first place, however.

Traditionally, much of the flavor that's added to food is in the form of fats and sugars, both of which are undesirable in a healthy lifestyle. With the help of friends who are chefs, I've succeeded in cutting down the quantities of fats and sugars I use. Better still, I've managed to eliminate them altogether in some cases. Instead, I flavor dishes with herbs and spices, using them either on their own or in combination.

As to whether the herbs should be fresh, dried, or frozen, I prefer fresh, especially when it comes to herbs like basil, tarragon, mint, and thyme, which I use regularly. Just in case they aren't available fresh at the store when I need them, I do have supplies of some dried herbs. Look for the kind that have been air dried because they retain the freshest flavor.

Organization is crucial – **time restraints** are one of the major reasons people **fail** in their attempts to follow **a diet plan.**

week 1

My key words of advice in this first important week are, 'don't overdo it.' Stay entirely in line with the plan. Do all that you're supposed to, no more and no less. You are about to make a fundamental change to your health and your appearance. Relax and enjoy it – this is an exciting time.

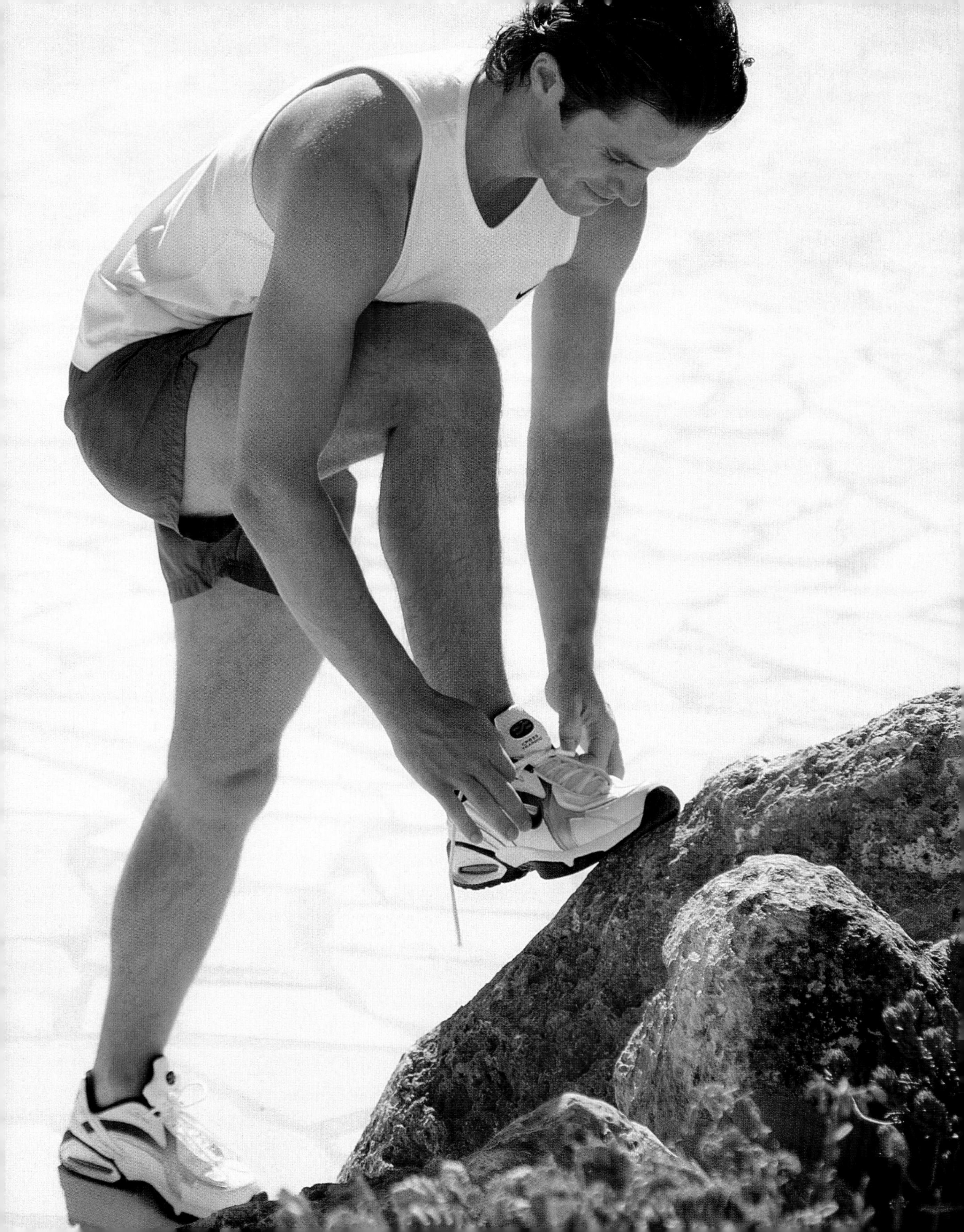

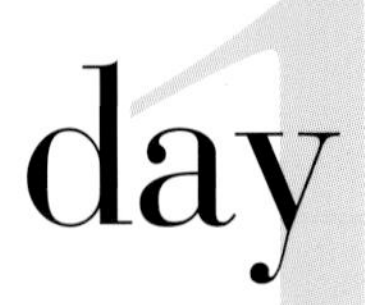

day 1

My goal today is to reactivate your body, to make you work muscles and joints that have been underused for too long. Your goal is to stick to the plan. If you can get through this first week, having completed all the workouts and having followed the diet plan to the letter, then week two will be easier for you to achieve.

Your first workout has three parts. The cardio is a 25-minute fast-pace walk. Walking at a steady pace keeps your heart rate within a small working zone – a technique called constant-pace training, which is crucial both for turning your body into an efficient fat-burner and for a good base level of fitness. Monitor how you're feeling. Be honest about it – that way you'll be able to measure your future success.

Move straight on to the resistance work and pay close attention to your technique. Finish the workout by performing a total body stretch.

eat&drink

breakfast wheat-free muesli *p132* **or** oatmeal *p132*

lunch smoked salmon sandwich *p139* **or** salade niçoise *p137*

dinner Asian stir fry *p141* **or** broiled fish with sweet potato and spinach bake *p144*

snacks banana, ½ oz (10 g) almonds, 2 oz (50 g) grapes **and** (for men) apple, and 4 oz (100 g) raspberries or 1 oz (25 g) raisins

drink at least 2½–3½ pints (1.5–2 liters) of water. And, remember, no more alcohol from now on

which fitness level?

If you scored fewer than 35 points in the fitness and nutrition test on pages 14–15, follow level ① in the resistance program on the opposite page. If you scored 35 points or more, follow level ②.

three-part workout

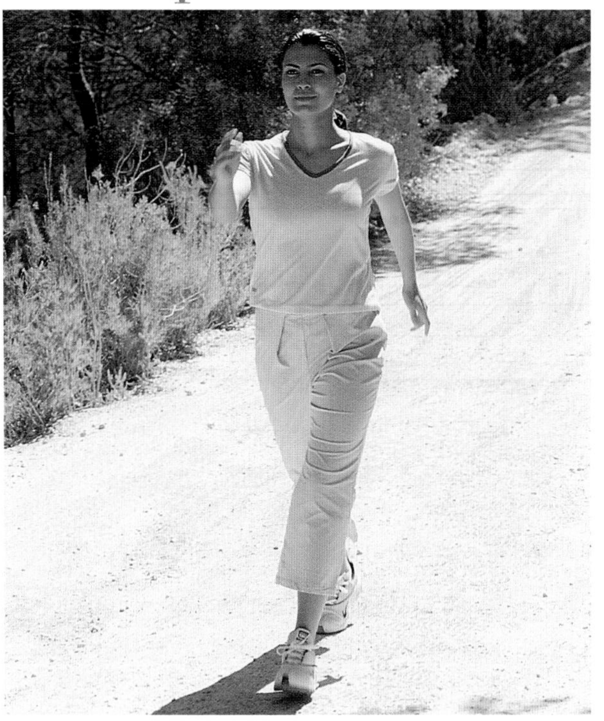

1 cardio

The cardio work today is a 25-minute fast-pace walk (the technique is explained on page 45). Enjoy it.

2 resistance

Your first program begins with the squat. Perform the number of reps (*p19*) indicated for your fitness level, rest for 30 seconds, and then repeat. Rest again for 30 seconds, and then move on to the body raise. Do this twice (with rests), and then do the same with the other exercises. With the glute raise, switch legs after your first set of 'reps,' so you work both legs. This approach to resistance is called 'working by sets.'

3 stretching

End the workout with a total body stretch sequence (*p22*). This should ward off soreness and stiffness in your muscles.

day 1 resistance work

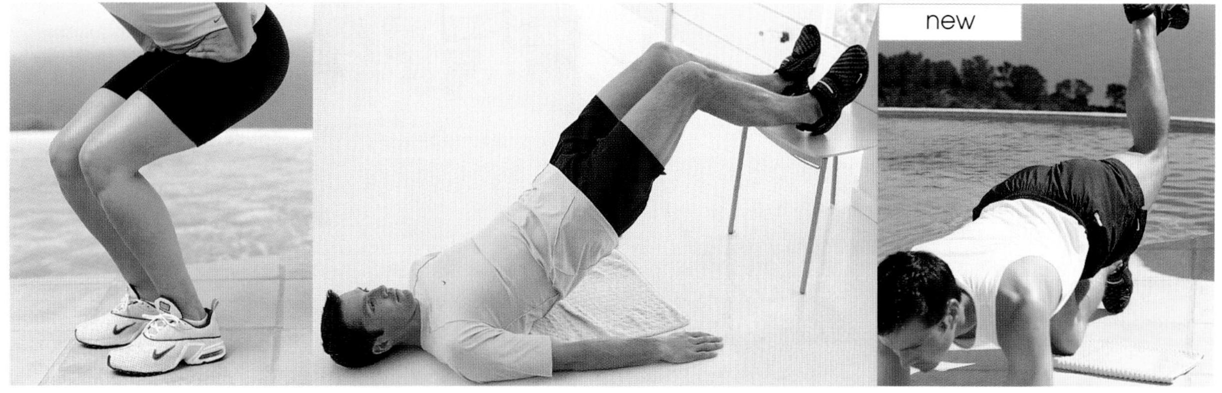

squat *p20*

① 15 reps ② 25 reps x2

body raise *p20*

① 15 reps ② 25 reps x2

glute raise *p38*

① 15 per leg ② 25 per leg x2

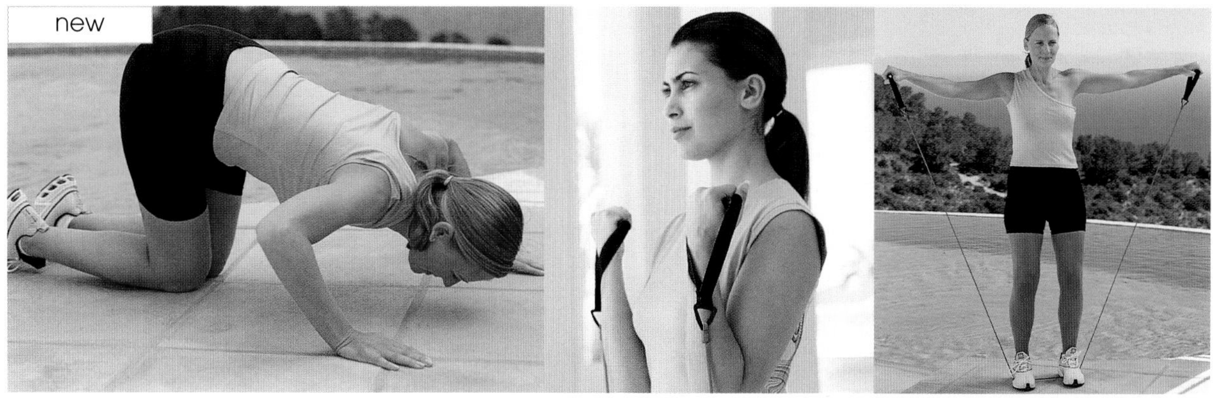

box push-up *p38*

① 15 reps ② 20 reps x2

bicep curl *p21*

① 12 reps ② 15 reps x2

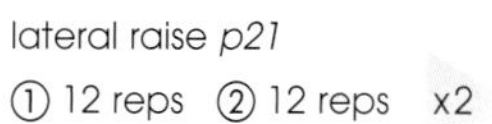

lateral raise *p21*

① 12 reps ② 12 reps x2

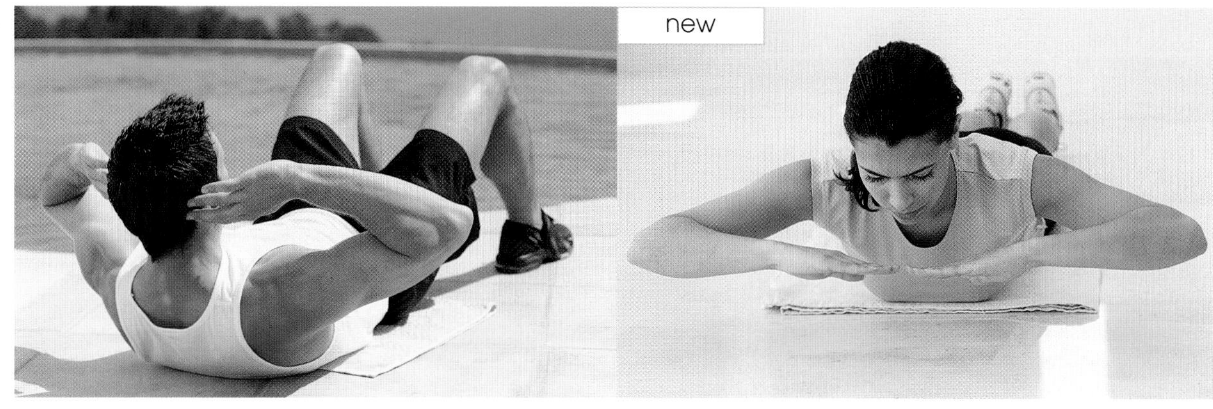

crunch *p21*

① 20 reps ② 30 reps x2

back extension *p38*

① 15 reps ② 20 reps x2

day 1 new exercises

glute raise ▷

Excellent for sculpting the largest muscle in your body – your bottom (glutes).

1 Support yourself on your forearms and knees, with your hands clasped together in front of you. Try to keep your back straight.

2 Raise one leg behind you as high in the air as you can. Keeping your knee bent and your foot flat, press up into the heel. Hold the position briefly, squeezing your buttocks, then slowly lower your leg to the start position.

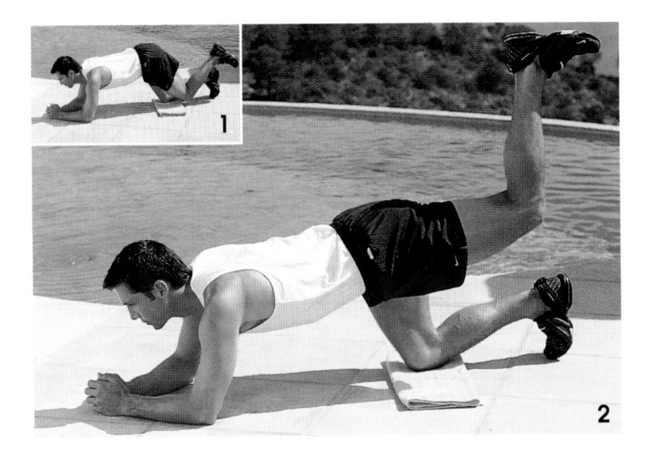

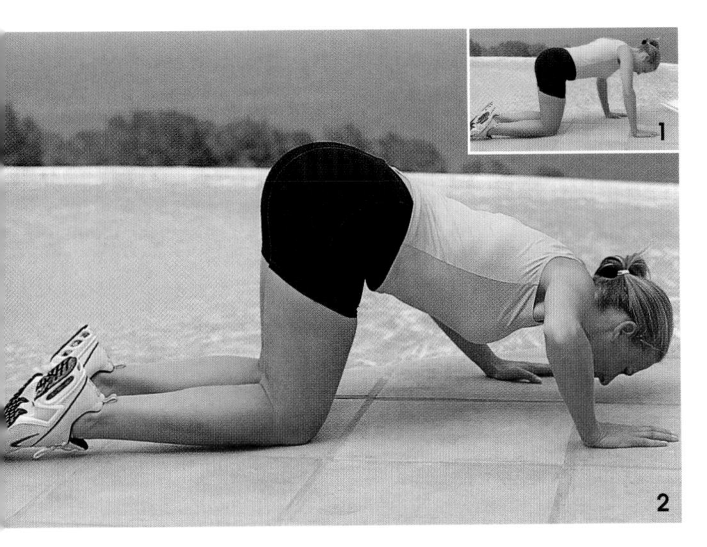

box push-up ◁

Great for giving you good 'T-shirt arms,' the box push-up is your first step toward the 'full' push-up.

1 Kneel on the floor with your knees directly under your hips. Place your hands slightly wider than shoulder-width apart under your shoulders. Make sure your fingers point forward. Keep your body weight over your hands, your tummy pulled in, and your back flat.

2 Keeping your body weight over your hands and maintaining a straight line through your torso, lower your body down so your elbows move to 90°. Push yourself back up to the start position.

back extension ▷

Good posture and 'core strength' (*p96*) come from both the front and back of the body. This exercise concentrates on strengthening your back.

1 Lie on your front and position your hands – fingertips touching – just above the floor under your chin.

2 Breathe out and at the same time raise your head and upper body off the floor, taking care not to tense your neck muscles. Hold for 1 second, then breathe in as you lower yourself. Keep the movement slow and controlled.

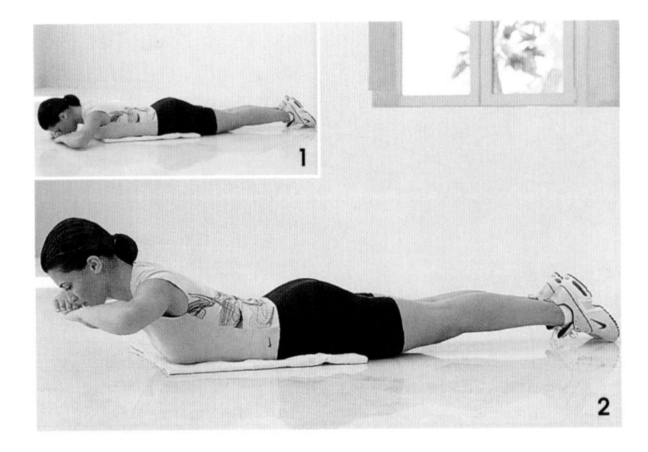

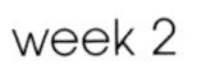

day 2

Even those of you who've never really exercised much before know that cardio exercise – like the fast-pace walking you did yesterday – makes you sweat. And that drinking water after exercising replenishes your body's fluid levels. It quenches your thirst, too, of course.

Today is your first rest day and you'll be pleased to hear I won't be asking you to build up a sweat. But I would like you to keep an eye on the amount of water you drink. My recommended daily intake is 2½–3½ pints (1.5–2 liters) of tap water or still mineral water every day (that doesn't include water in coffee, tea, sweetened fruit juices, and carbonated drinks, by the way). It may seem like a lot to some of you, but drinking plenty of water really does help your body function more efficiently. It can even help you shed weight, too, as your body flushes out fluids it's been retaining.

eat&drink

breakfast fresh fruit salad with yogurt and seeds *p132* **or** two slices of whole-wheat toast with nonhydrogenated spread (*see p32*) and jam or jelly

lunch wild rice salad *p136* **or** quinoa salad *p136*

dinner polenta-crusted swordfish with sweet potato *p145* **or** wheat-free pasta with tomato and shrimp sauce *p148*

snacks apple, pear, 1 oz (25 g) sunflower seeds, 1 oz (25 g) raisins **and** (for men) banana, 1 oz (25 g) sunflower seeds, ½ oz (10 g) raisins

drink at least 2½–3½ pints (1.5–2 liters) of water

▷ In general, good healthy food should make up 80% of your diet. While you're following the fat loss plan, however, it will make up 100%. The food may be low in calories, but I haven't stinted on the flavor, I can assure you of that.

The **good news** is that your **rest days** are almost as **important** as your exercise days, so **make the most of them.** Don't feel guilty about **chilling** today.

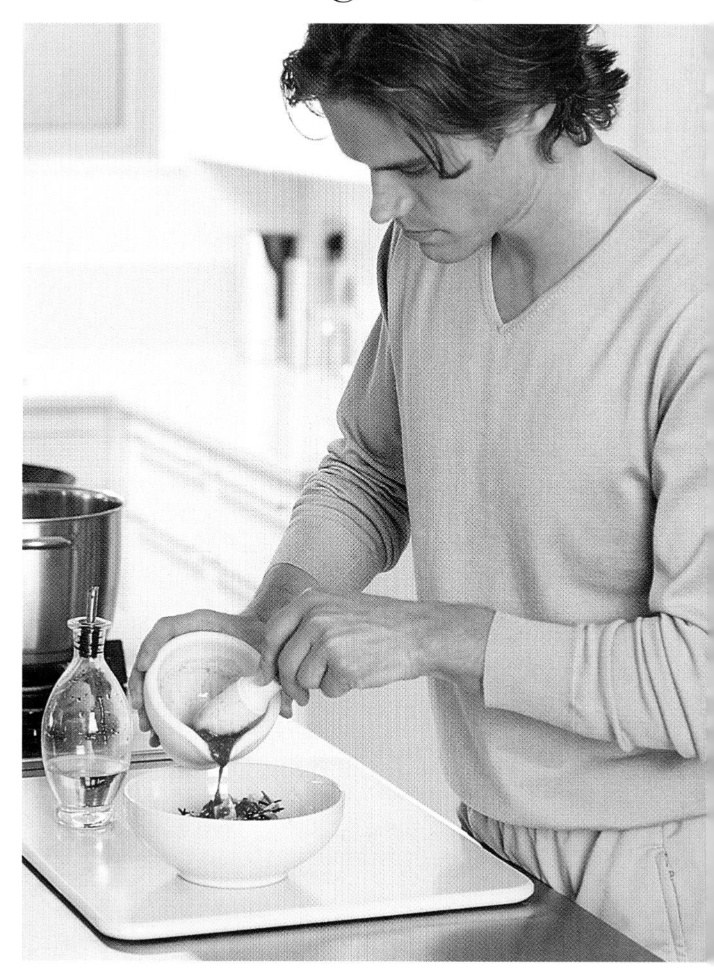

day 3

Each week, I'll ask you to repeat a workout you've done before. Today is the first time that happens – you'll repeat day 1. Aim to give the same level of commitment to today's work as you did then.

eat & drink

breakfast wheat-free muesli *p132* **or** poached egg on two slices of dry whole-wheat toast

lunch asparagus and artichoke salad *p135* **or** Greek salad *p134*

dinner sweet potato gnocchi with tomato and shrimp sauce *p140* **or** chicken and vegetable kabobs *p143*

snacks apple, pear, and 4 oz (100 g) raspberries or 1 oz (25 g) dried apricots **and** (for men) 1 oz (25 g) mixed sunflower and sesame seeds, 1 oz (25 g) raisins

drink at least 2½–3½ pints (1.5–2 liters) of water

three-part workout

As you perform your 25-minute fast-pace walk today, remember you're aiming to burn fat. This means working within your optimum training zone, which today should be 70% of your maximum heart rate (MHR). Before you set off for your walk, refresh in your mind the theory of MHR (*p17*) and check page 156, where I give you the heart rate in beats per minute that you should be working at. Make sure you know how to take your pulse (*p17*), too.

When you've walked for 5 minutes, stop to take your pulse. Calculate your heart rate and then compare it with the rate I recommend. You may need to increase or decrease your pace accordingly. Check your MHR again after 5 minutes to make sure you're getting the pace right.

Move on to repeat day one's resistance work and then finish your workout with a total body stretch (*p22*).

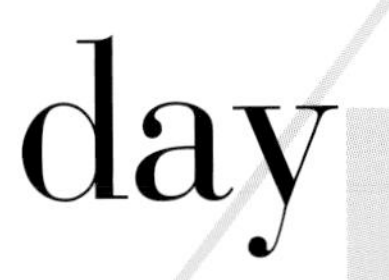

day 4

This is a rest day, so there's no workout for you to perform. Try to spend a little time making sure you've established in your mind your goal for the next eight weeks. Remember, you really need to know what your dream is before you can make it come true. Start keeping a diary. Write down your goal, and then record how you're getting on with your workouts and diet plan each day.

Quite often it helps to talk things through with a friend, a member of your family, or a colleague – whoever you think will be most supportive. Highlight areas you think you'll have to work hardest in and where you'll need most encouragement. If the person you've chosen is the positive influence you think they are, you could be pleasantly surprised by how much they'll be prepared to do to keep you on course with the plan.

One word of warning: beware of those people who are eager to tell you about their own past failures, or who suggest more effective diets or better workouts. Stay focused on this, your fat loss plan, and keep your personal goal in sight.

eat & drink

breakfast fresh fruit salad with yogurt and seeds *p132* **or** vegetable omelet *p133*

lunch salade niçoise *p137* **or** broiled vegetable pitas *p139*

dinner Thai-style vegetables with polenta *p141* **or** steamed cod with green lentils and tomatoes *p147*

snacks banana, ½ oz (10 g) almonds, 2 oz (50 g) grapes **and** (for men) apple, and 4 oz (100 g) raspberries or 1 oz (25 g) raisins

drink at least 2½–3½ pints (1.5–2 liters) of water

5 day

By now, you may be feeling a bit stiff after your first couple of workouts. It's possible, too, that you're a little hungry and missing your regular foods. You are making progress, however, and starting to lose fat, so take a positive attitude into your day today. There's a new resistance program for you to do.

As the days go by and you try different workouts and different dishes, you'll probably find you discover your likes and dislikes. Certain exercises become a lot easier and more enjoyable as you get fitter, and you might just surprise yourself how much you are adjusting to the change in diet.

eat&drink

breakfast fresh fruit salad with yogurt and seeds *p132* **or** wheat-free muesli *p132*

lunch beet and carrot salad *p134* **or** green salad *p134*

dinner chicken with couscous and mint yogurt *p149* **or** carrot and sweet potato fishcakes with herb salad *p144*

snacks apple, pear, 1 oz (25 g) sunflower seeds, 1 oz (25 g) raisins **and** (for men) banana, 1 oz (25 g) sunflower seeds, ½ oz (10 g) raisins

drink at least 2½–3½ pints (1.5–2 liters) of water

three-part workout

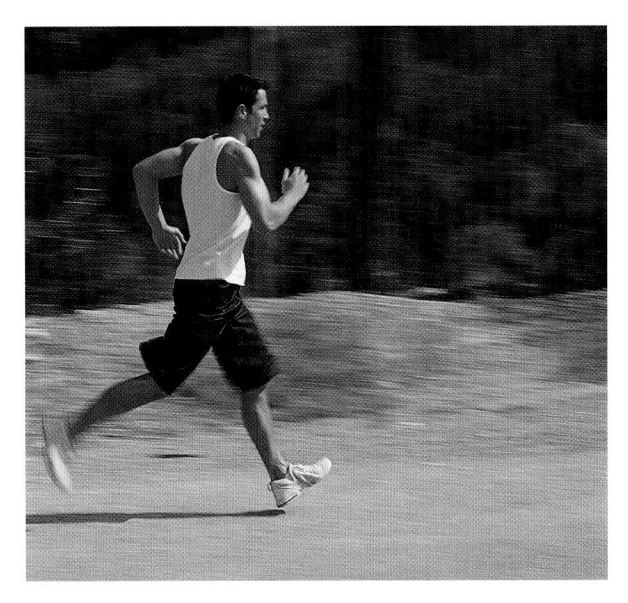

1 cardio

Today, I'd like you to fast-pace walk or run (*p77*) for 30 minutes. This is 5 minutes more than before and will increase the session's impact. Work at 70% MHR (*see day 3*).

2 resistance

The squat and the body raise are your first two exercises again, but I've modified the 'set' work. Start with the set of squat reps, rest for 30 seconds, then do the body raise reps. Rest, then repeat the squat reps and then the body raise reps. Rest again, then perform one last set of both.

Now move on to the abductor raise reps. Rest, then continue with the glute raise reps. Perform a set of both once more, with a rest in between.

Finally, perform the crunch reps, the back extension reps, and the reverse curl reps in that order twice, with a 30-second rest between each set of reps.

3 stretching

Finish your workout with a lower body stretch (*p23*).

day 5 resistance work

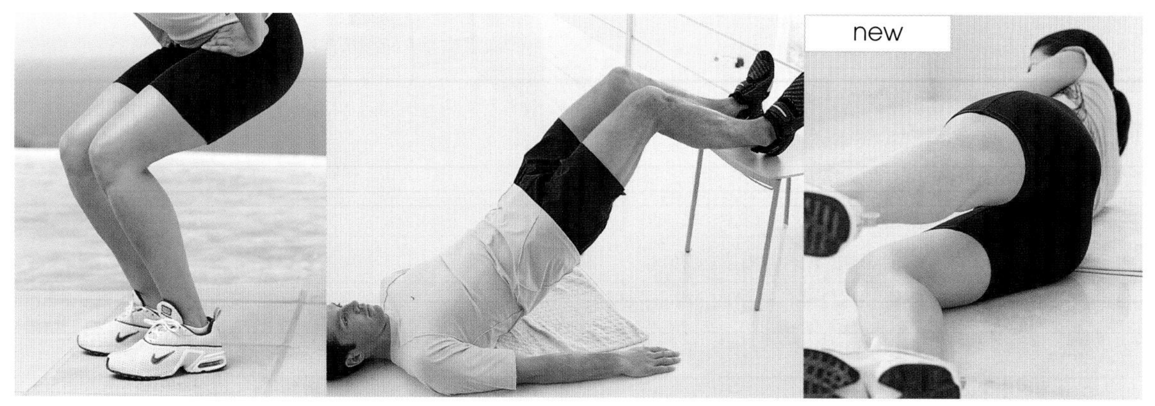

squat *p20*
① 15 reps ② 25 reps

body raise *p20*
① 15 reps ② 25 reps x3

abductor raise *p43*
① 20 reps per leg ② 25 reps per leg

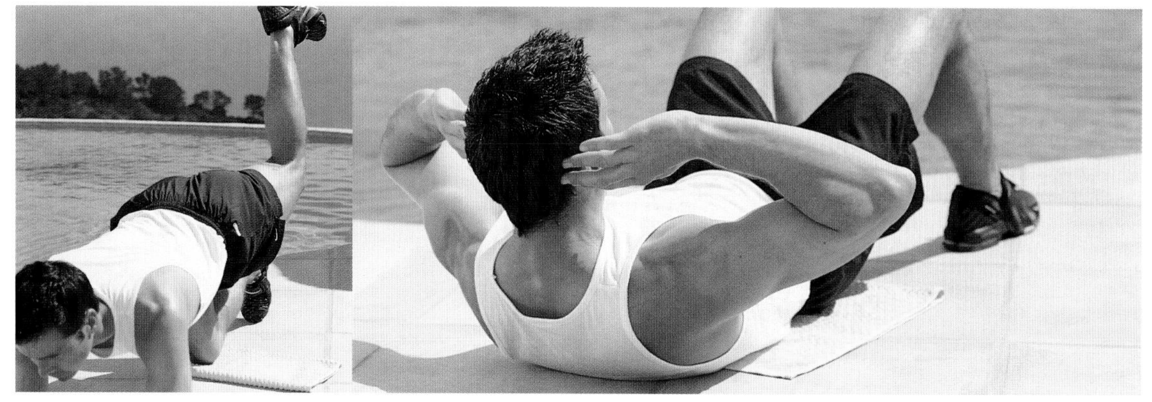

glute raise *p38*
① 18 per leg ② 25 per leg x2

crunch *p21*
① 20 reps ② 40 reps

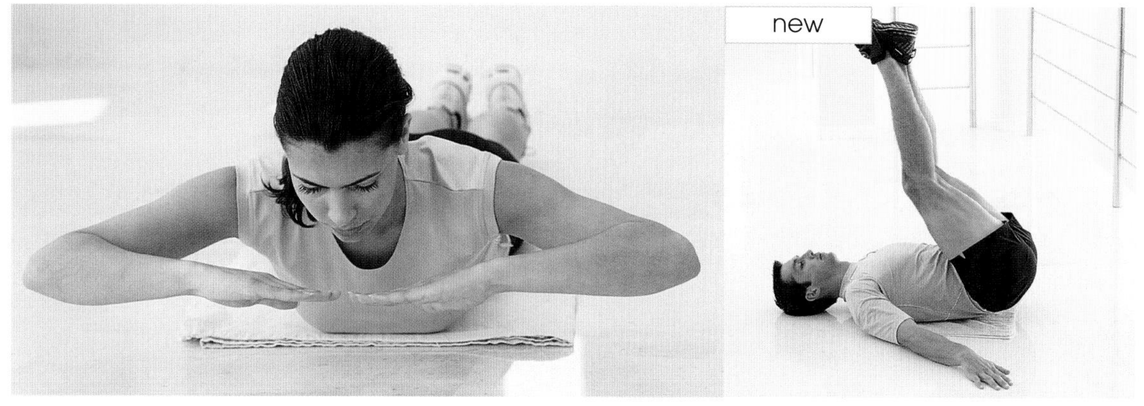

back extension *p38*
① 15 reps ② 20 reps

reverse curl *p43*
① 12 reps ② 20 reps x2

day 5 new exercises

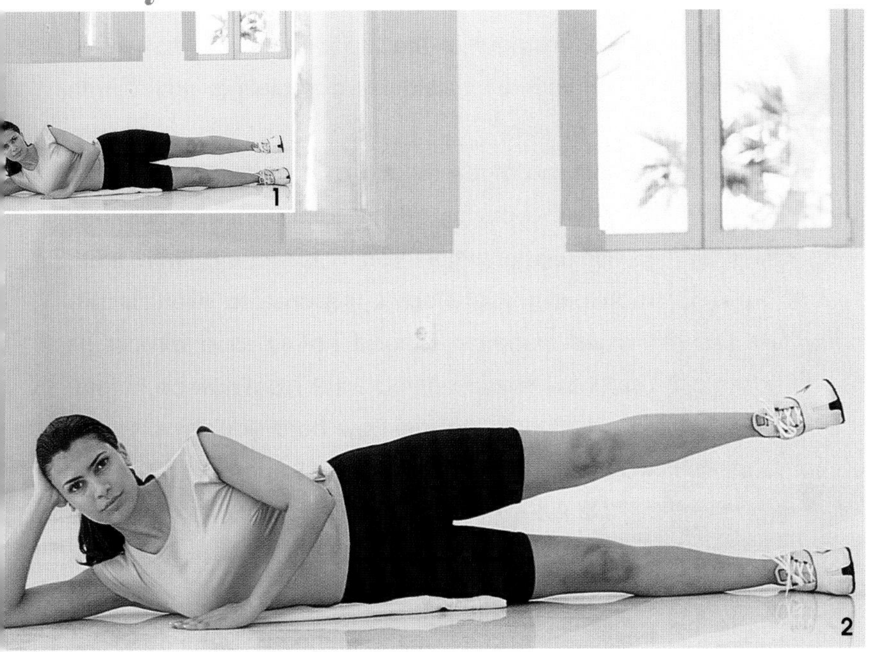

abductor raise ◁

This shapes your hips and the top of your buttocks to make you look longer and narrower.

1 Lie on your side with your lower leg slightly bent. Use the hand of your lower arm to support your head, and place the hand of your upper arm in front of you to steady yourself.

2 Breathe in. Keeping your upper leg straight and in line with your body, lift it up with a slow, controlled movement. Hold for 1 second, then slowly lower your leg to the start position, breathing out as you do so.

reverse curl ▷

For good strong tummy muscles, you need to do several exercises, among them the reverse curl. Performed in conjunction with other 'crunches,' it tones your stomach from the lower part up.

1 Lie on your back, with your arms out to the sides, your palms to the floor, and your legs straight up in the air. Keep your head and shoulders on the floor at all times and make sure your feet never come farther back than your head.

2 Breathe in, then tighten your lower tummy muscles and bring your legs and pelvis back toward your rib cage. Keep the movement slow and controlled, never allowing your legs to swing around. Hold for 1 second, then slowly lower your legs to the floor, breathing out as you do so.

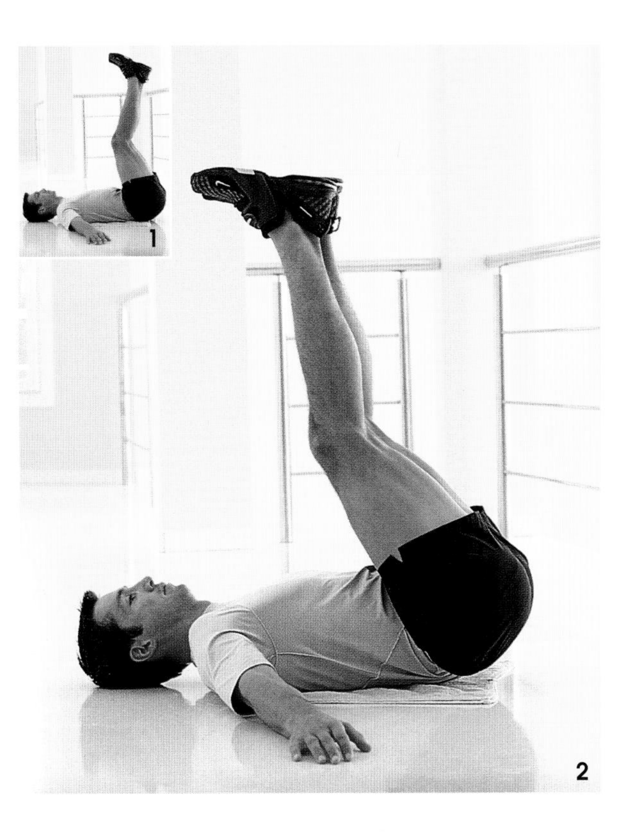

day 6

Breakfast is the most important meal of the day, and should always be substantial enough to last you through to lunchtime (apart from a strategic snack somewhere in the middle of the morning, that is). For those of you who really can't face eating too much first thing in the morning – even on a rest day, when you don't have to work out – a smoothie is ideal. It's quick to make, easy to digest, and gives your body the boost it needs, when it most needs it.

eat&drink

breakfast a small fruit smoothie *p133* and two slices of whole-wheat toast with nonhydrogenated spread and jam or jelly **or** oatmeal *p132* and a piece of fruit

lunch wild rice salad *p136* **or** tuna sandwich *p138*

dinner stuffed bell pepper *p142* **or** broiled fish with sweet potato and spinach bake *p144*

snacks apple, pear, and 4 oz (100 g) raspberries or 1 oz (25 g) dried apricots **and** (for men) 1 oz (25 g) mixed sunflower and sesame seeds, 1 oz (25 g) raisins

drink at least 2½–3½ pints (1.5–2 liters) of water

a smoothie gives your body a boost when it needs it most – first thing in the morning.

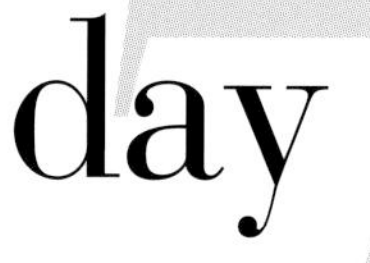

day 7

You've made it to the last day of your first week. Make yourself proud by completing day 7 with flying colors.

You should be feeling as if you've made some progress – your breathing, for instance, should feel a little easier when you're exercising. With time, monitoring your body's response to exercise like this will become second nature, and almost as useful as measuring your MHR. From now on, in fact, I'll ask you to gauge how hard you think you're working and match it to an RPE number.

The RPE (rate of perceived exertion) scale is a convenient way of calculating how hard you're working. Many people find it easier than taking their pulse and doing the arithmetic required to get their MHR. During today's cardio, work at level 7, which means you should be breathless and a bit sweaty. The complete scale is on page 157.

eat&drink

breakfast whole-wheat pancakes *p132* **or** oatmeal *p132*

lunch quinoa salad *p136* **or** Greek salad *p134*

dinner salmon and vegetable kabobs *p143* **or** wheat-free pasta with tomato and shrimp sauce *p148*

snacks banana, ½ oz (10 g) almonds, 2 oz (50 g) grapes **and** (for men) apple, and 4 oz (100 g) raspberries or 1 oz (25 g) raisins

drink at least 2½–3½ pints (1.5–2 liters) of water

three-part workout

Today is a straight repeat of day 5, even down to your choice of cardio. Finish with a lower body stretch (*p23*).

the best fast-pace walking technique

Fast-pace walking is one of the best ways of burning fat and keeping fit. It's also low impact. Here are my eight top tips for your technique.

- ▸ Walk with your chin up and look forward.
- ▸ Keep your neck and shoulders relaxed.
- ▸ As you step forward, plant your heel first, then roll through with your body weight. At the same time, bring your front hand up to chest height.
- ▸ When your body weight is on your front foot, push your back leg into the stride (you should be able to feel your buttock and thigh muscles working). Pull your other arm back strongly as you do so.
- ▸ Hold your tummy muscles tight.
- ▸ Don't overstride – keep your stride length short.
- ▸ Keep your hips square and facing forward.
- ▸ Breathe deeply from your stomach if you can.

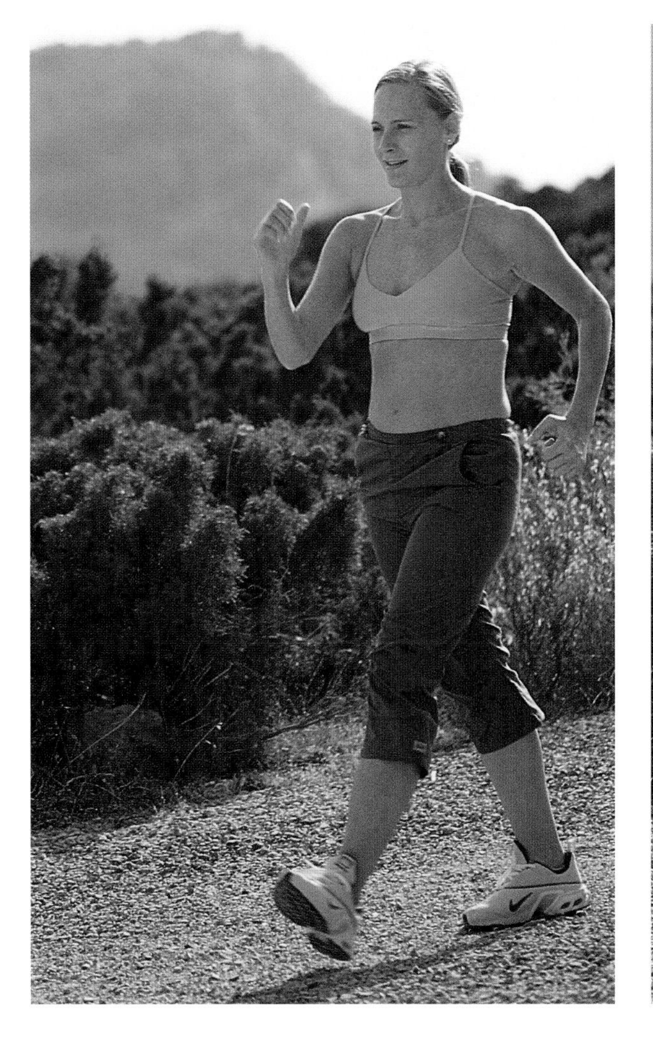

▽ To step forward, plant your front heel on the ground, then roll your body weight through. Only when you've transferred your weight should the back leg begin to push.

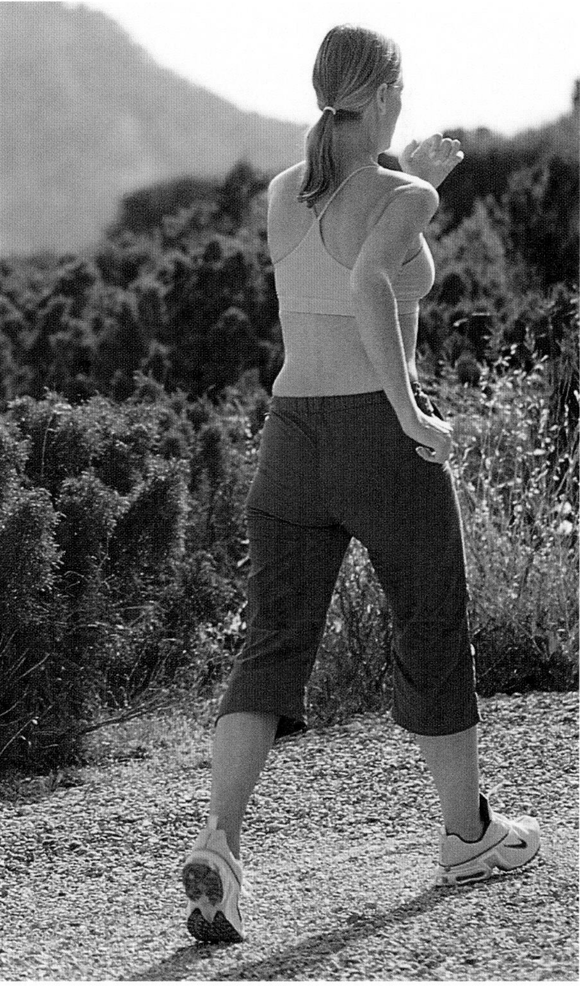

▽ Powering you forward, your buttocks are the workhorses of fast-pace walking. This is the reason that walking makes your bottom look lean and trim.

week 2

At this stage, my clients usually feel as if they're about to explode – they're itching to go farther and faster. Despite a bit of stiffness and tiredness, you're probably feeling the same right now. Your motivation is high and you're focused on achieving your goals. So keep right on track. Stick to the plan. And keep making the changes. You're doing well.

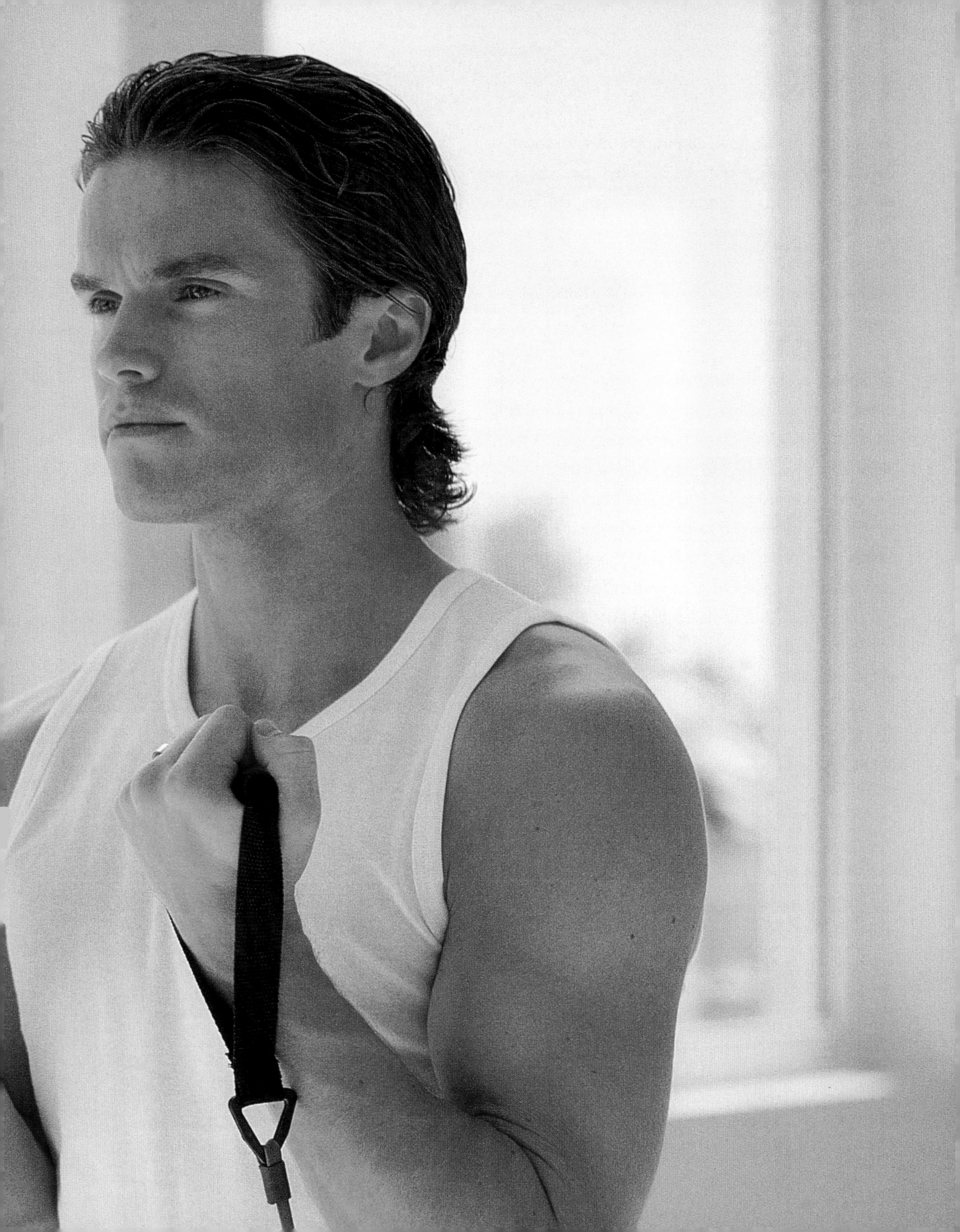

day 8

As you go about your day-to-day business today, spend some time thinking about ways to make your life more active. It could help you reach your goals.

I've mentioned your basal metabolic rate (BMR) before. This is the rate at which your body burns calories. The cardio exercise you're doing at the moment is excellent for raising your BMR.

Research shows, however, that it's often a person's daily activity level that makes the difference between losing weight and retaining it. So any chance you have of increasing your activity level is worth seizing. The opportunities abound.

Modern living makes us quite lazy, but it's easy to bypass many labor-saving devices. You can climb the stairs instead of taking the elevator. You can make a short journey on foot rather than taking the car or bus. And by doing these things, you speed up your metabolic rate. I'll give you more ideas later in the plan. In the meantime, keep your BMR in mind.

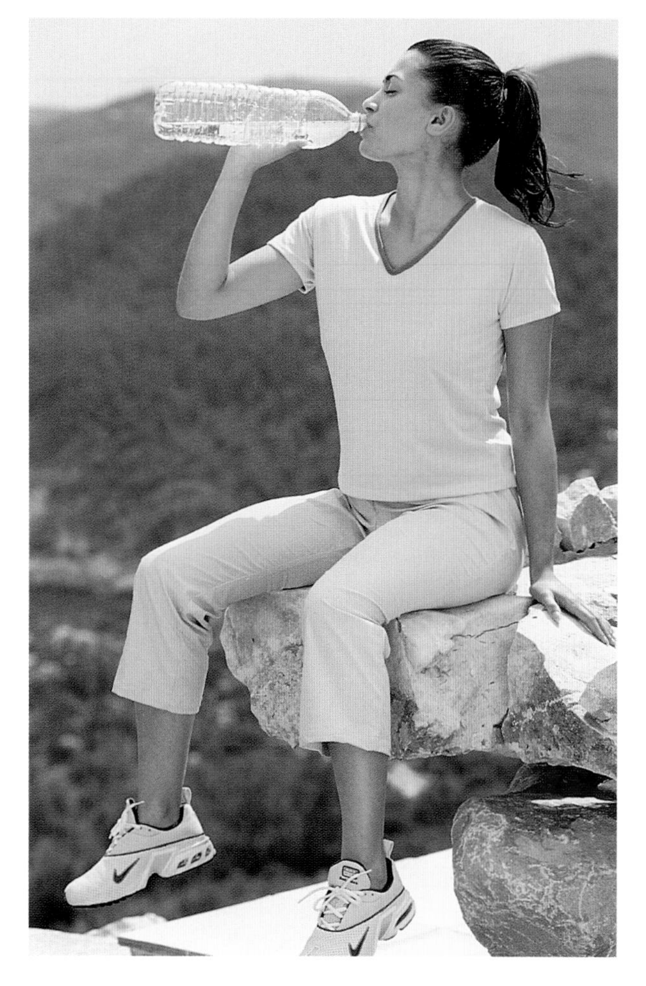

△ Before, during, and after – that's my message where exercise and drinking water are concerned. Aim to have a glassful every 10 minutes when you're working out.

eat&drink

breakfast fresh fruit salad with yogurt and seeds *p132* **or** two slices of whole-wheat toast with nonhydrogenated spread and jam or jelly

lunch broiled vegetable pitas *p139* **or** smoked salmon and dill salad *p138*

dinner monkfish with roasted vegetables *p146* **or** Asian stir fry *p141*

snacks apple, pear, 1 oz (25 g) sunflower seeds, 1 oz (25 g) raisins **and** (for men) banana, 1 oz (25 g) sunflower seeds, ½ oz (10 g) raisins

drink at least 2½–3½ pints (1.5–2 liters) of water

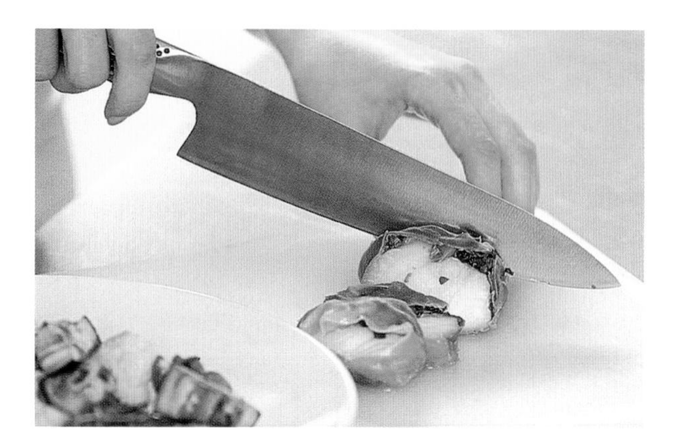

▷ A rest day is a great opportunity to prepare a special dinner, such as monkfish with roasted vegetables.

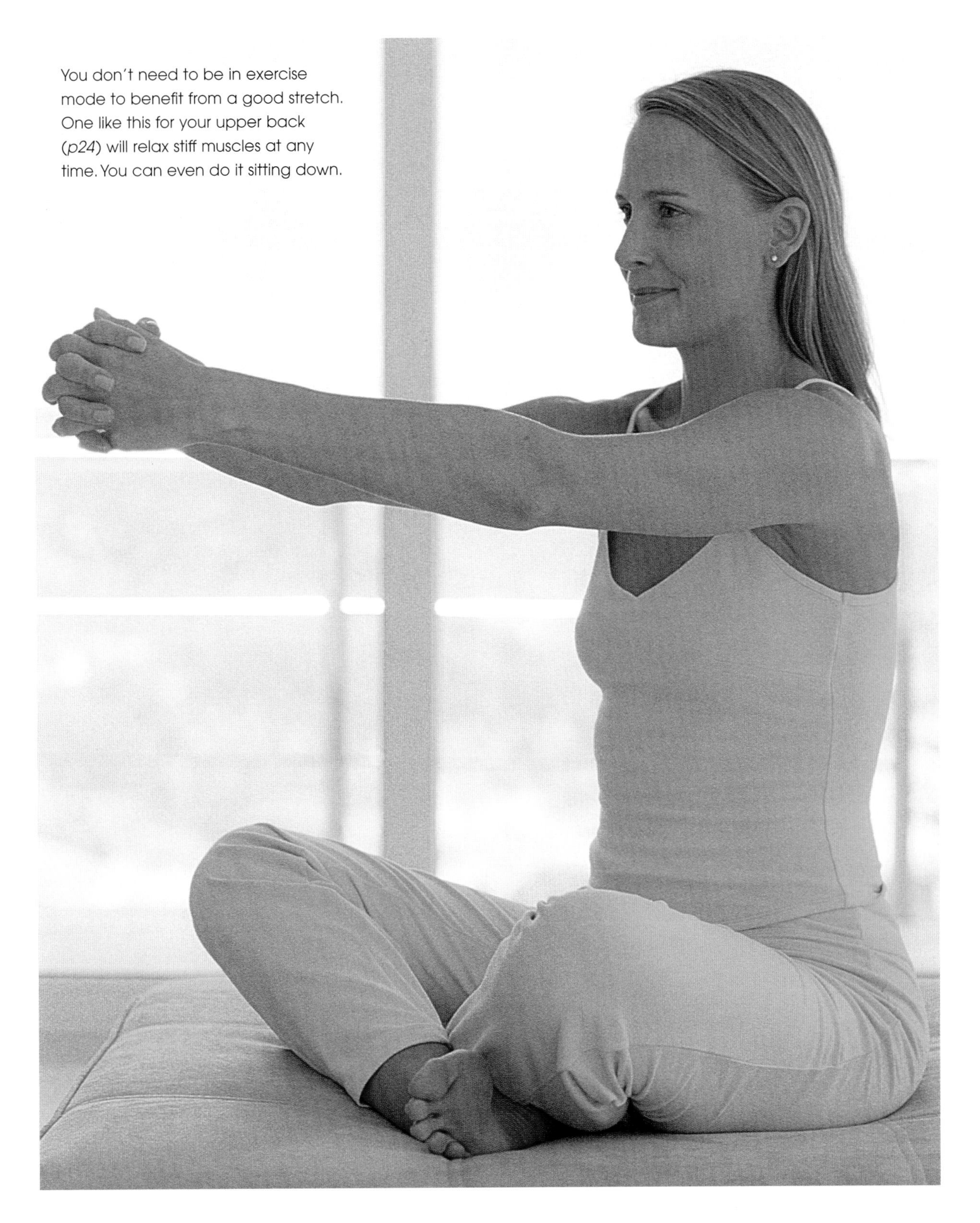

You don't need to be in exercise mode to benefit from a good stretch. One like this for your upper back (*p24*) will relax stiff muscles at any time. You can even do it sitting down.

day 9

It's time to step things up: you've had just over a week to get into the plan and your body is starting to adjust. This next week you'll see big changes.

eat&drink

breakfast wheat-free muesli *p132* **or** vegetable omelet *p133*

lunch beet and carrot salad *p134* **or** shrimp and linguine salad *p137*

dinner smoked salmon and lentil salad *p147* **or** mushroom risotto *p142*

snacks apple, pear, and 4 oz (100 g) raspberries or 1 oz (25 g) dried apricots **and** (for men) 1 oz (25 g) mixed sunflower and sesame seeds, 1 oz (25 g) raisins

drink at least 2½–3½ pints (1.5–2 liters) of water

three-part workout

1 cardio

As you do your cardio today, you'll be taking your heart rate up and down in intensity (a fat-burning technique called interval training). Start by fast-pace walking for 2 minutes, then run for 2 minutes at 80% MHR (8/10 RPE). Repeat seven times (so you walk and run eight times in all).

2 resistance

Perform the exercises with 10-second rests in between, then repeat twice. Level ② users, increase the resistance on your exertube (by wrapping the cord around your feet, say). You're doing fewer reps than level ①, but working harder.

3 stretching

Finish today's workout with a total body stretch (*p22*).

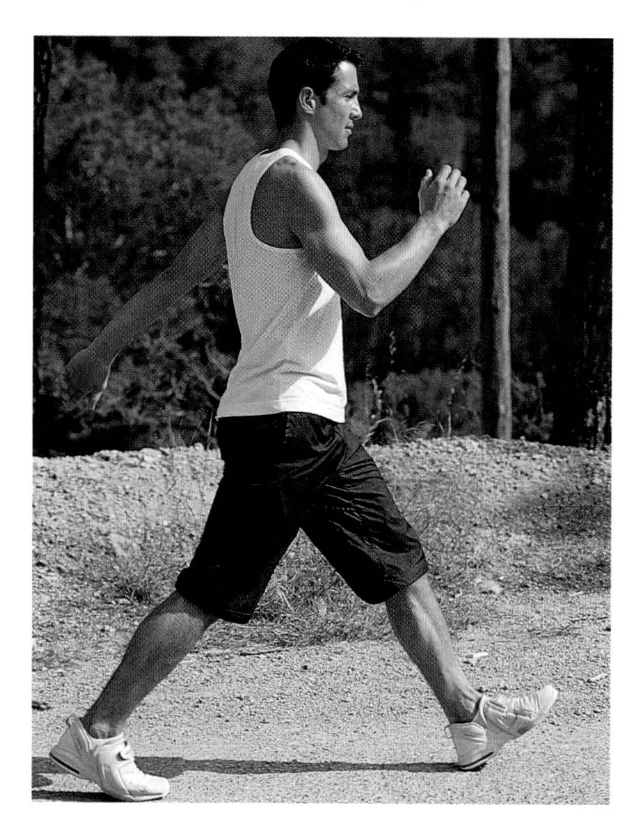

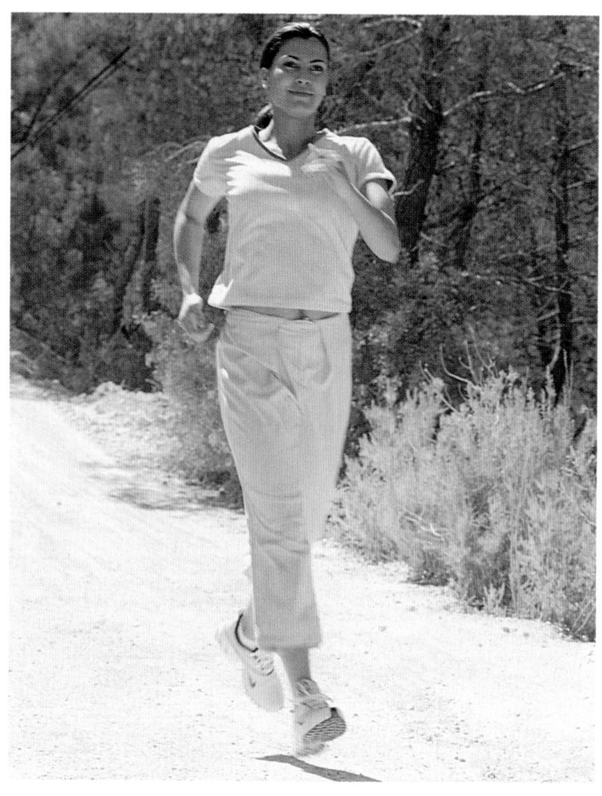

day 9 resistance work

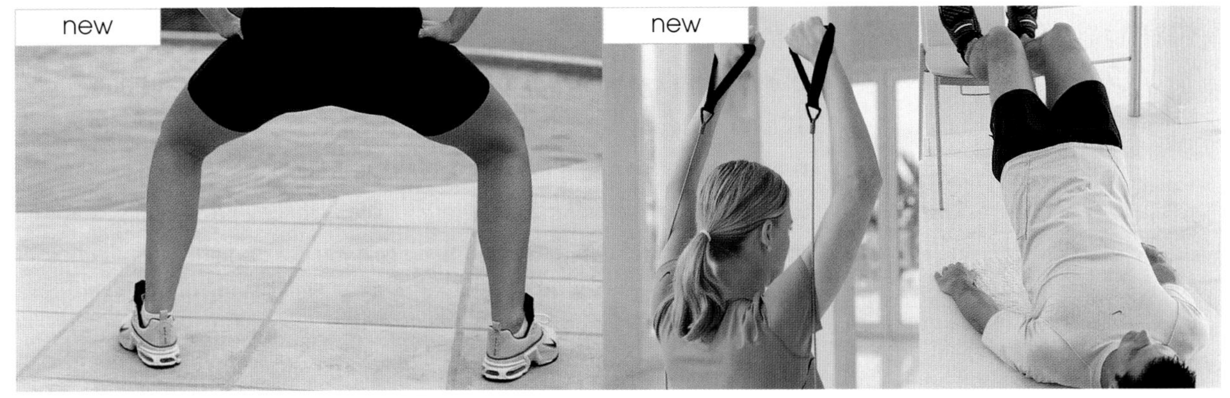

wide squat *p52*
① 15 reps ② 25 reps

shoulder press *p52*
① 15 reps ② 15 reps

body raise *p20*
① 15 reps ② 25 reps

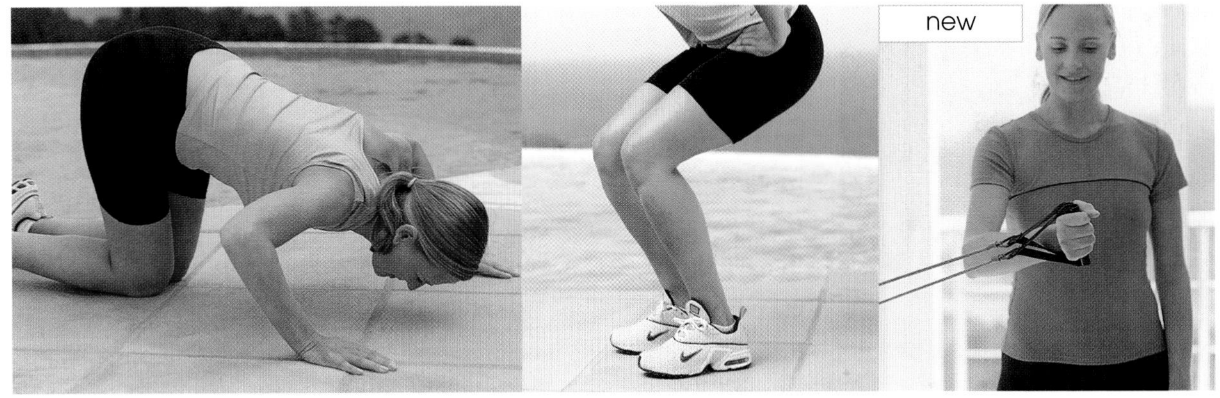

box push-up *p38*
① 15 reps ② 25 reps

squat *p20*
① 20 reps ② 25 reps

pec fly *p52*
① 15 reps per arm ② 12 reps per arm

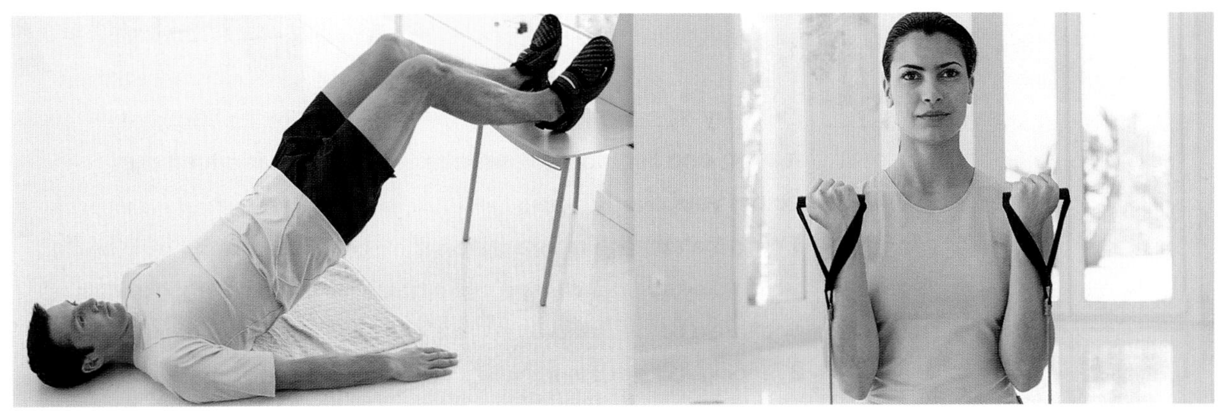

body raise *p20*
① 15 reps ② 25 reps

bicep curl *p21*
① 15 reps ② 12 reps x3

day 9 new exercises

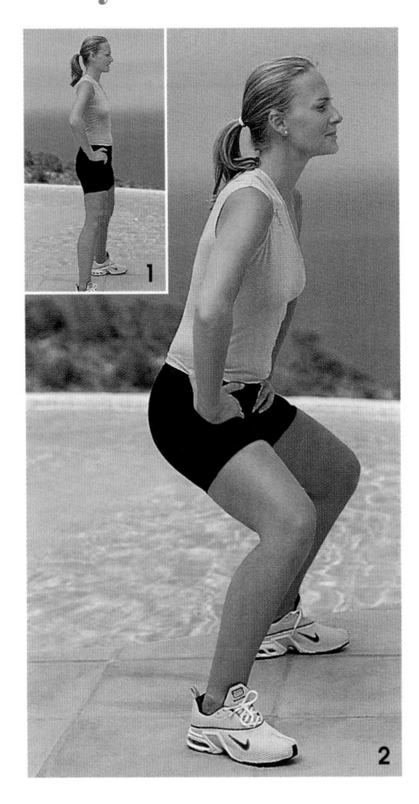

wide squat ◁

Like the 'basic' squat, but tougher on your inner thighs and butt.

1 Stand with your feet slightly wider than shoulder-width apart and your toes pointing out at an angle. Place your hands on your hips.

2 Keeping your feet still and bending your knees so they travel over your toes (but not beyond them), lower your body as if you are about to sit on a chair. When you're 'sitting' just above 90°, slowly raise your body to the start.

shoulder press ▷

To define upper arms, so you look good in a sleeveless top.

1 Place your feet hip-width apart in the middle of the exertube, knees slightly bent. With a handle in each hand, raise your arms so your elbows are at 90° at shoulder height.

2 Push your hands up until your arms are almost fully extended above your shoulders. Keep a slight bend in your elbows. Lower your arms to the start.

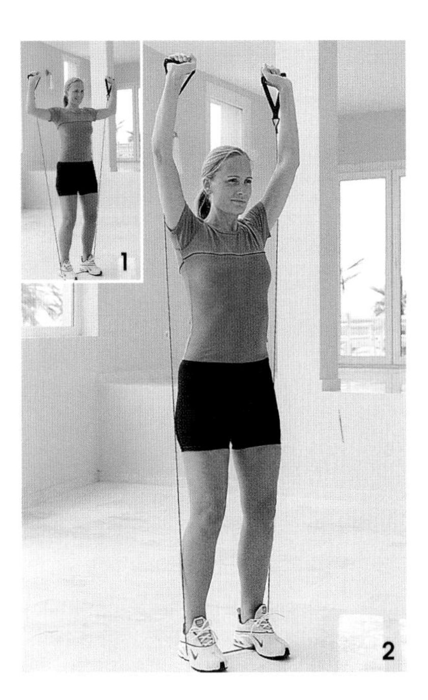

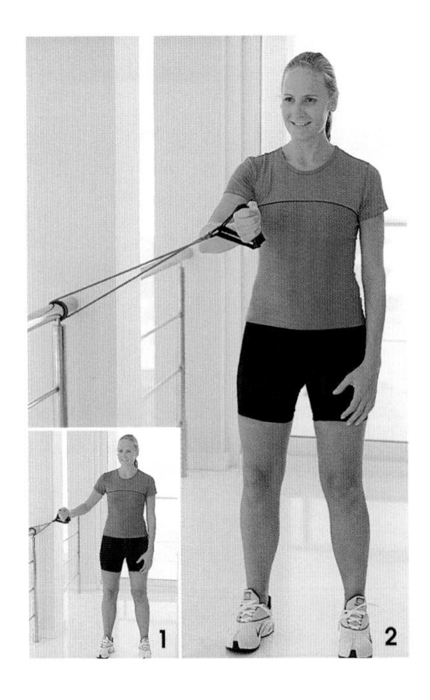

pec fly ◁

A lifting and firming exercise that gives you muscle tone right across your chest (pecs).

1 Wrap the exertube around a strong pole or handle at about waist height. Stand sideways just under arm's-length from the pole, your legs hip-width apart. Hold both exertube handles in one hand, arm slightly bent.

2 Keeping your shoulders and legs completely static and your elbow slightly bent, bring your hand around toward you so the handles of the exertube are directly in front of your chest. Slowly return to the start position.

day 10

You're making great strides forward, so today you can have a breather before two consecutive days of exercise. Taking it easy (or easier!) on your rest days is vital. But it's just as important to eat well. To recover properly from its exertions, your body needs to be fed correctly. And when you come to work it, it needs to have the best 'fuel' you can supply it with. Make sure you're doing the very best for your body – and yourself – by eating the right foods in the right quantities. Stick closely to the diet plan I've worked out for you.

eat & drink

breakfast oatmeal *p132* **or** wheat-free muesli *p132*

lunch asparagus and artichoke salad *p135* **or** salade niçoise *p137*

dinner broiled or steamed fish with quinoa *p143* **or** lemon shrimp with three bean salad *p148*

snacks banana, ½ oz (10 g) almonds, 2 oz (50 g) grapes **and** (for men) apple, and 4 oz (100 g) raspberries or 1 oz (25 g) raisins

drink at least 2½–3½ pints (1.5–2 liters) of water

Make sure you do the very best for your body – and yourself. Stick closely to the diet plan and you'll soon see results.

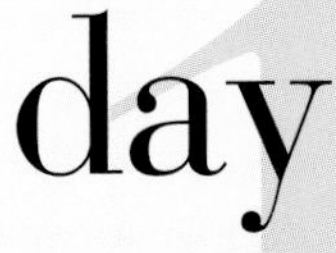

day 11

There are a few days – like today – when I'll ask you to do a two-part workout only. These are your 'cardio only' days or your 'resistance only' days, and the beauty of them is that you can give your all to the session and be finished in just over 40 minutes. Make every effort to push yourself 100%, though.

eat & drink

breakfast whole-wheat pancakes *p132* **or** two slices of whole-wheat toast with nonhydrogenated spread and jam or jelly

lunch wild rice salad *p136* **or** Camargue rice salad *p136*

dinner smoked salmon and lentil salad *p147* **or** carrot and sweet potato fishcakes with herb salad *p144*

snacks apple, pear, 1 oz (25 g) sunflower seeds, 1 oz (25 g) raisins **and** (for men) banana, 1 oz (25 g) sunflower seeds, ½ oz (10 g) raisins

drink at least 2½–3½ pints (1.5–2 liters) of water

two-part workout

For the cardio part of the workout, run or walk at a constant pace for 40 minutes. Work at 75% MHR (7–8/10 RPE). There's no resistance work today, so finish the workout by performing a lower body stretch (*p23*).

day 12

In an ideal world, we'd be able to give ourselves completely to every part of every workout. In reality, though, this just doesn't work. So today, focus your energy on the resistance part of your workout. Your muscles have had a few days off from being worked intensively, so they should have recovered from any stiffness and be raring to go.

eat&drink

breakfast fresh fruit salad with yogurt and seeds *p132* **or** large fruit smoothie *p133*

lunch broccoli salad *p135* **or** cottage cheese, cranberry and arugula sandwich *p138*

dinner vegetable and tofu kabobs with rice *p143* **or** monkfish with roasted vegetables *p146*

snacks apple, pear, and 4 oz (100 g) raspberries or 1 oz (25 g) dried apricots **and** (for men) 1 oz (25 g) mixed sunflower and sesame seeds, 1 oz (25 g) raisins

drink at least 2½–3½ pints (1.5–2 liters) of water

Focus your energies **on** your **resistance** work today. Your muscles have had time to **recover** from any stiffness, so they should be **raring to go.**

three-part workout

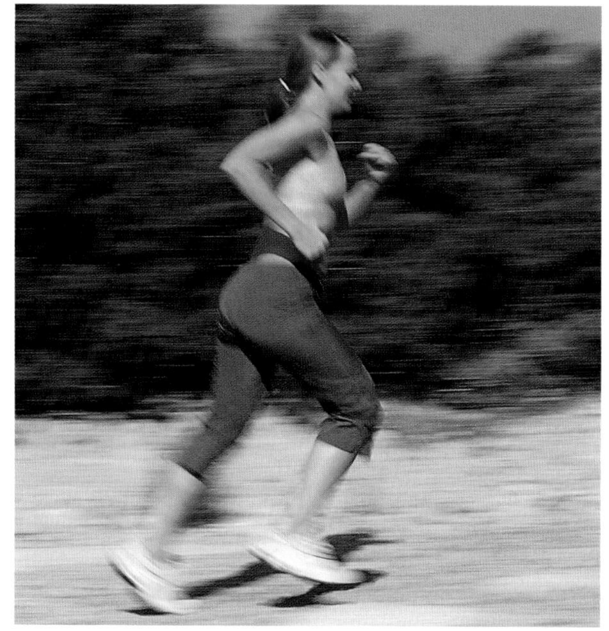

1 cardio

Run or walk at a constant pace for 40 minutes. Work at 75% MHR (7–8/10 RPE). If you can, push yourself a little harder than you did yesterday (although you may feel it's already much harder today because you're a bit tired).

2 resistance

The approach to today's resistance work is the same as that on day 9 – the exercises alternate between those for your upper body and those for your lower body. It's a training technique called peripheral heart action (PHA), which works your body harder and burns more fat. Do all the exercises in order, rest for 2 minutes, then repeat.

3 stretching

End today's workout with a total body stretch (*p22*).

day 12 resistance work

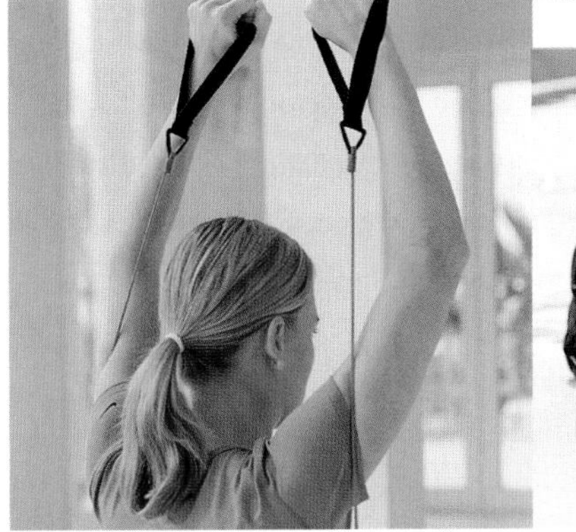

shoulder press *p52*

① 15 reps ② 20 reps

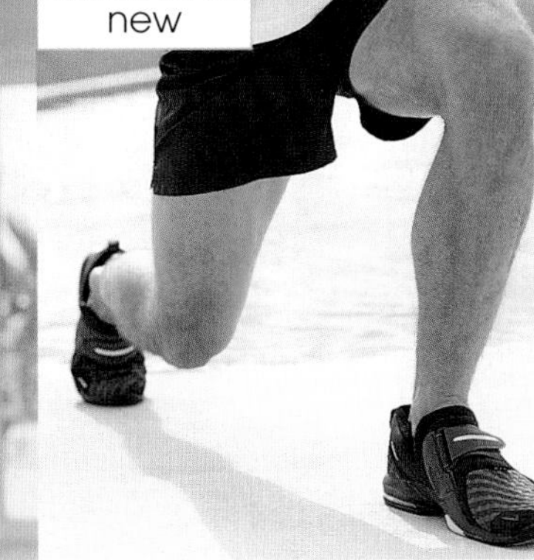

lunge *p56*

① 15 reps per leg ② 20 reps per leg

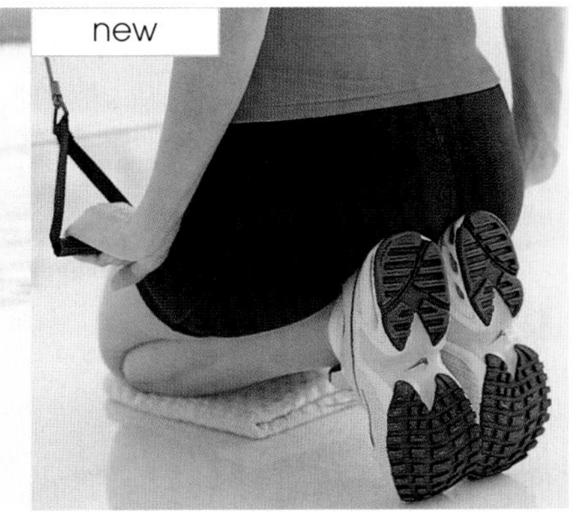

tricep press *p56*

① 15 reps ② 15 reps

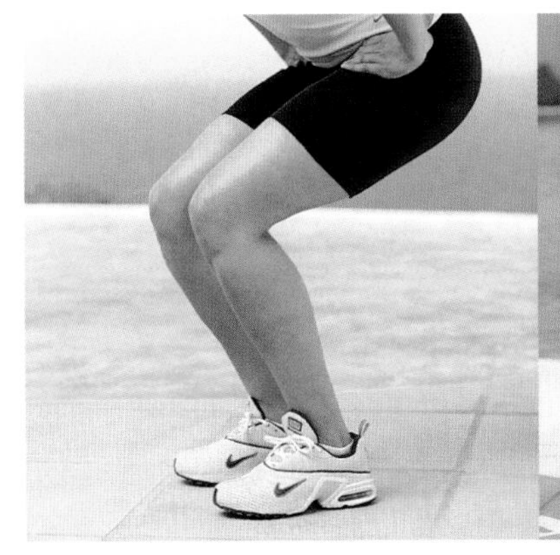

squat *p20*

① 20 reps ② 25 reps

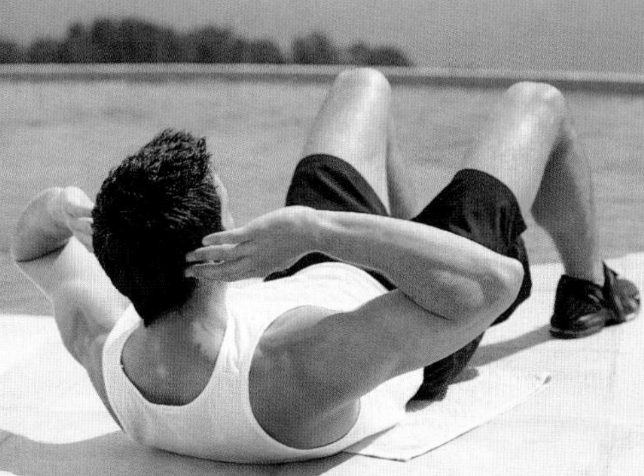

crunch *p21*

① 25 reps ② 30 reps

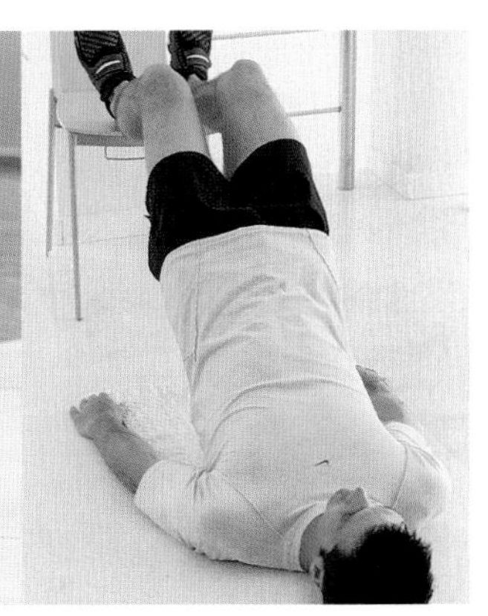

body raise *p20*

① 20 reps ② 20 reps

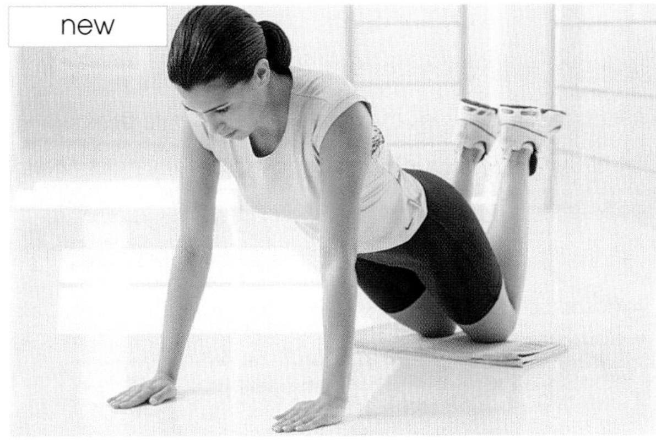

extended box push-up *p56*

① 15 reps ② 25 reps

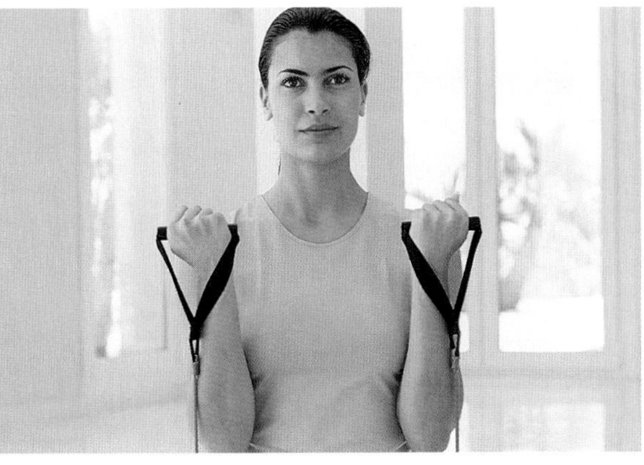

bicep curl *p21*

① 15 reps ② 15 reps x2

day 12 new exercises

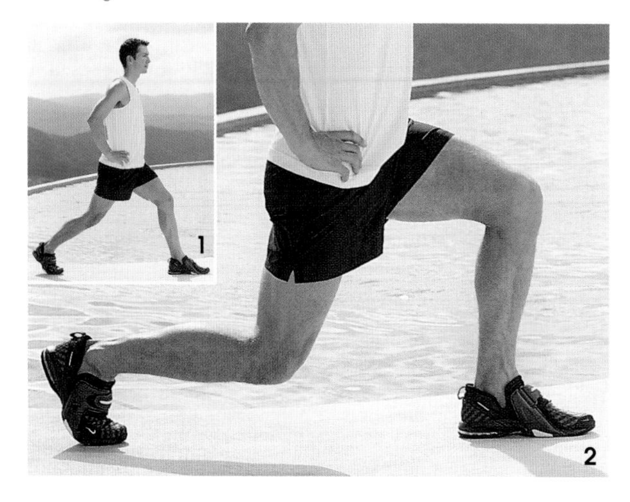

lunge ◁

Possibly the most effective way to work your lower body muscles, particularly your thighs and buttocks.

1 Place one foot in front of you about one stride-length from your back foot. Keep your hips facing straight ahead and your hands on your hips. Keep your body upright and your tummy muscles pulled in.

2 Bend your knees to bring your front knee directly over your front foot. Put your weight on the heel of your front foot to maximize the work on the muscle of your buttock. Slowly return to the start position.

tricep press ▷

This exercise targets the 'wobbly' bits behind your arms that you pretend aren't really there!

1 Wrap the exertube around a strong pole or handle at about eye level. Place a mat on the floor at arm's-length from the pole. Kneel on the mat with your toes on the floor, then sit back on your heels. Keep your back straight and your tummy pulled in. Hold the exertube handles in both hands. Keep your palms facing downward and your elbows tucked in tight.

2 Keeping your elbows tucked in, push both arms down until they're fully extended. Keep your back straight and your tummy muscles pulled in. Slowly raise your arms to the start position.

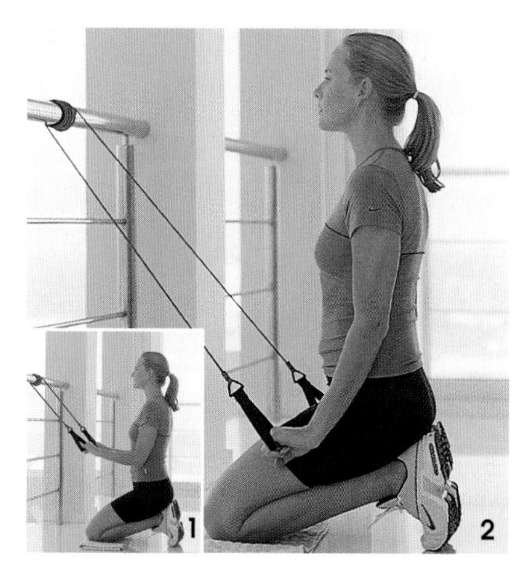

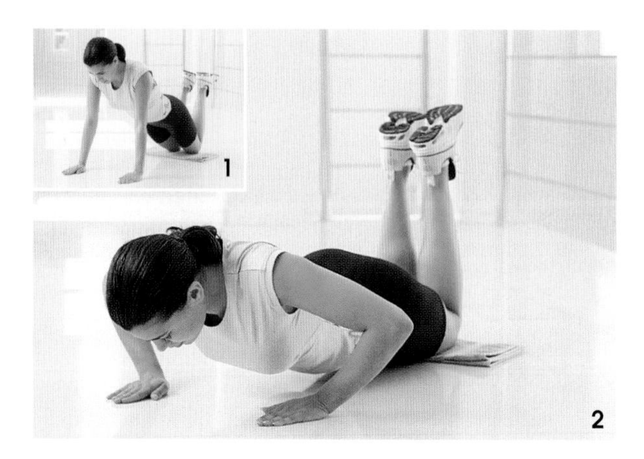

extended box push-up ◁

A harder version of the push-up, this puts extra pressure on your upper arms, shoulders, and chest.

1 Kneel with your knees directly under your hips. Place your hands slightly wider than shoulder-width apart under your shoulders, and raise your lower legs to 90°. Keep your fingers pointing forward and your head facing down.

2 Keeping your weight over your hands and maintaining a straight line through your torso, lower your body down so your elbows move to 90°. Slowly push back up to the start.

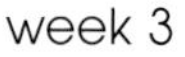

day 13

Whether you're superstitious or not, today is no day to risk making a mistake or falling behind schedule, so take the day off.

Seriously, though, there are times when you shouldn't exercise. If you're feeling exhausted or run down, or if you feel as if you're about to come down with a cold or the flu, it's wise to take a short break from working out. Your immune system will be working hard enough as it is without your depleting your body's vital reserves of energy by exercising vigorously. You run the risk of making the symptoms worse and your recovery more prolonged.

If at any time you feel faint or dizzy while you're working out, stop immediately – it could be that you're pushing your body too hard and it simply can't cope. Try to get into the sensible habit of checking your MHR as you exercise – that way you'll always know when you're working within your optimum training zone.

eat & drink

breakfast poached egg on two slices of dry whole-wheat toast **or** vegetable omelet *p133*

lunch Greek salad *p134* **or** quinoa salad *p136*

dinner marinated tuna with polenta *p145* **or** steamed cod with green lentils and tomatoes *p147*

snacks banana, ½ oz (10 g) almonds, 2 oz (50 g) grapes **and** (for men) apple, and 4 oz (100 g) raspberries or 1 oz (25 g) raisins

drink at least 2½–3½ pints (1.5–2 liters) of water

day 14

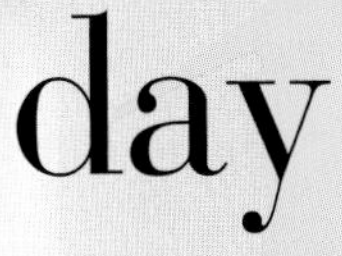

As you perform your cardio today, monitor how you're feeling. Think about your breathing and how your legs feel. And when you've finished the session, check how long it takes you to recover. Now think back to how you felt two weeks ago when you'd just started the plan.

Taking stock of your body's response to exercise like this means you're learning to listen to your body and how it feels. This is an enormous part of being fit and healthy.

eat & drink

breakfast wheat-free muesli *p132* **or** oatmeal *p132*

lunch smoked salmon and dill salad *p138* **or** beet and carrot salad *p134*

dinner wheat-free pasta with turkey *p148* **or** steamed fish with Moroccan vegetables *p146*

snacks apple, pear, 1 oz (25 g) sunflower seeds, 1 oz (25 g) raisins **and** (for men) banana, 1 oz (25 g) sunflower seeds, ½ oz (10 g) raisins

drink at least 2½–3½ pints (1.5–2 liters) of water

three-part workout

This is a repeat of day 12, but instead of performing exactly the same cardio work, either run or fast-pace walk today, whichever you didn't do two days ago. The change of activity will give your body a new challenge. Work for 40 minutes at 75% MHR (7–8/10 RPE).

Your resistance is the same PHA work. This will make your heart work harder as it increases the blood supply to the extremities of your body, so your resistance work will have an almost 'aerobic' feel.

Finish the workout with a total body stretch (*p22*).

week 3

It's happening! You're **losing weight**, getting fitter, and those **jeans are** definitely **feeling looser**. But you're **tired**, you can't wait to get into bed at night, and you're **missing** some of your usual **treats**. Surely, all this **hard work** means you can have one or two. No, it doesn't; that's how trouble starts. This is only week three and you have a lot to do. **Trust me.**

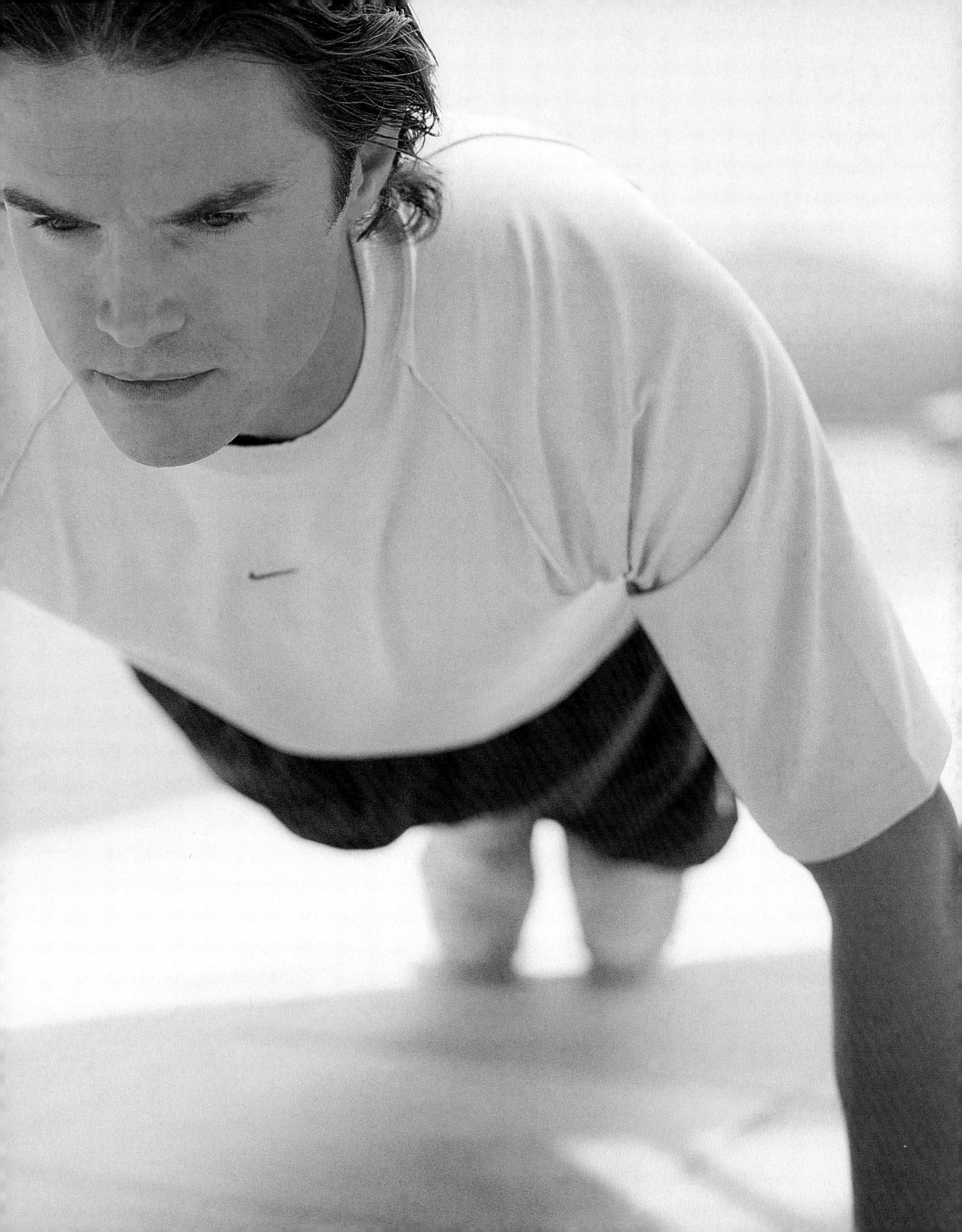

day 15

Now that your initial rush of excitement about the fat loss plan is beginning to fade, you're probably coming to the realization that you're in this for the long haul. Good! I'd like you to use this week as a test to see if you can maintain your discipline through what will be the toughest time for you.

I'm about to up your workload by giving you a new way to train. Compound training, as it's called, is all about growth, and will give you massive gains in strength. It will develop your muscles, but only enough to make them extremely active. If you feel them expanding, don't worry – it's only temporary and it will help you through the coming stages.

eat&drink

breakfast fresh fruit salad with yogurt and seeds *p132* **or** oatmeal *p132*

lunch shrimp and linguine salad *p137* **or** wild rice salad *p136*

dinner baked zucchini with rice *p140* **or** broiled or steamed fish with quinoa *p143*

snacks apple, pear, and 4 oz (100 g) raspberries or 1 oz (25 g) dried apricots **and** (for men) 1 oz (25 g) mixed sunflower and sesame seeds, 1 oz (25 g) raisins

drink at least 2½–3½ pints (1.5–2 liters) of water

three-part workout

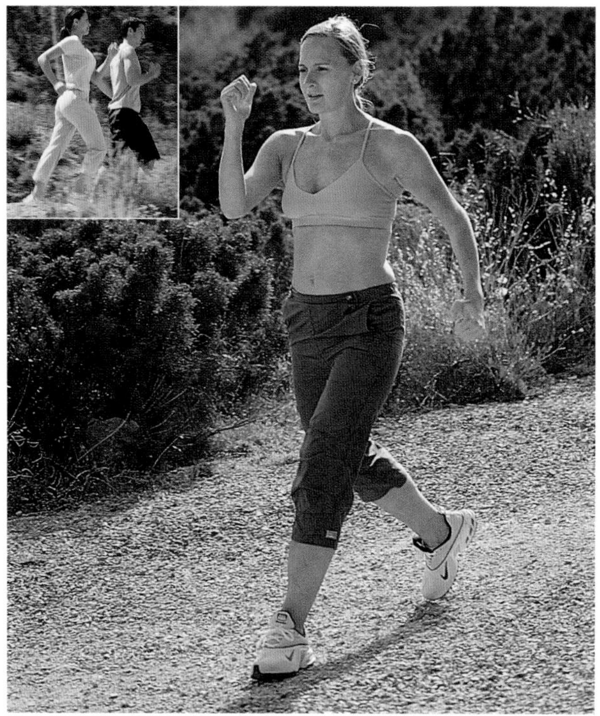

1 cardio

Fast-pace walk for 1 minute, then run for 1 minute. Repeat this 11 times (so you walk and run 12 times in all). Run at 85% MHR (8–9/10 RPE).

2 resistance

Today you'll start 'compound training,' which means working the same part of your body in different ways in back-to-back sets. In today's work, you start with your upper arms. Do the first three exercises. Repeat them, then rest for 2 minutes. Do the next two exercises, repeat twice, and then rest again. Finally, do the last three, rest for 2 minutes, and repeat. Level ② users, make sure you have plenty of resistance on your exertube (*see day 9*).

3 stretching

Finish today's workout with a total body stretch (*p22*).

day 15 resistance work

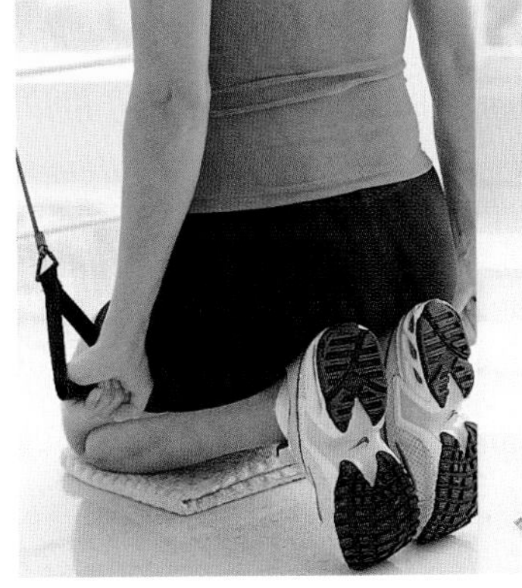

tricep press *p56*
① 12 reps ② 12 reps

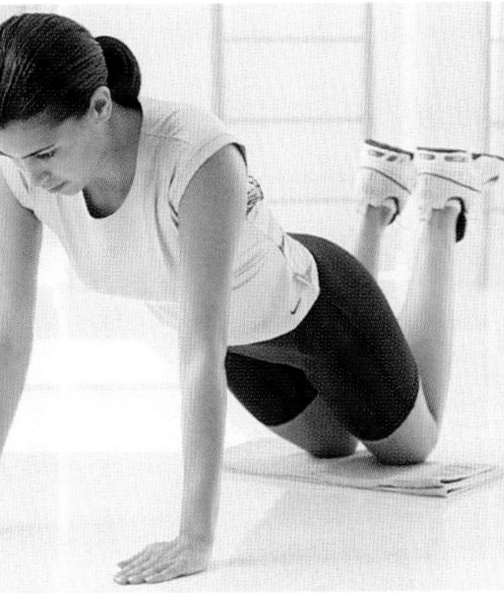

extended box push-up *p56*
① 20 reps ② 25 reps

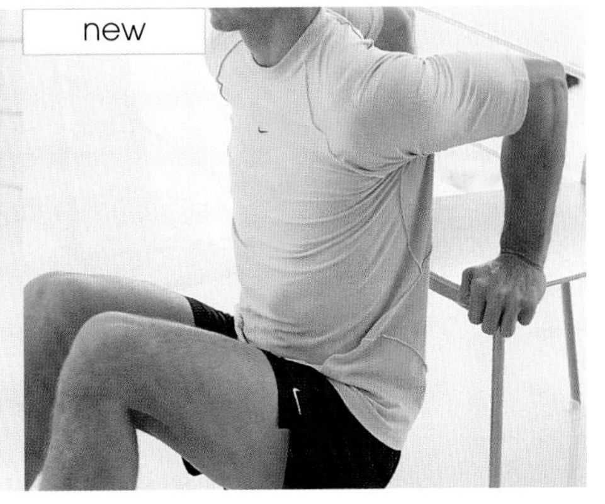

dip *p62*
① 20 reps ② 20 reps x2

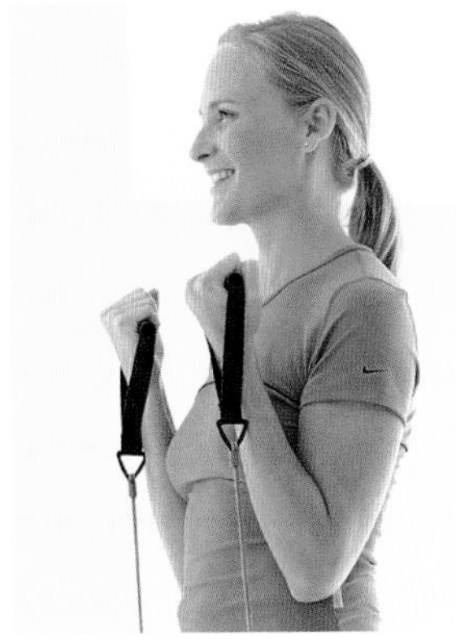

bicep curl *p21*
① 20 reps ② 15 reps

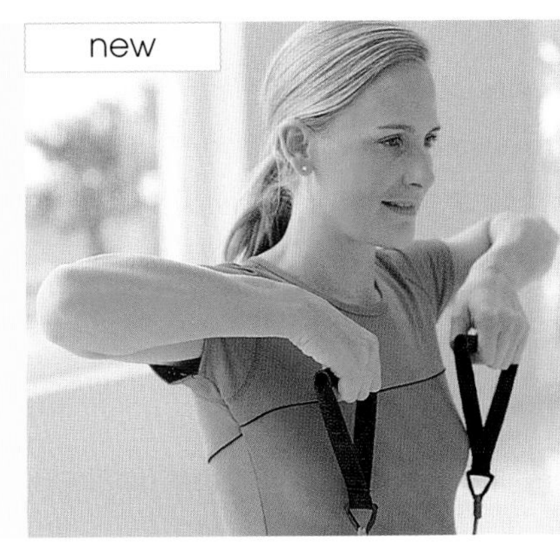

upright row *p62*
① 20 reps ② 15 reps x3

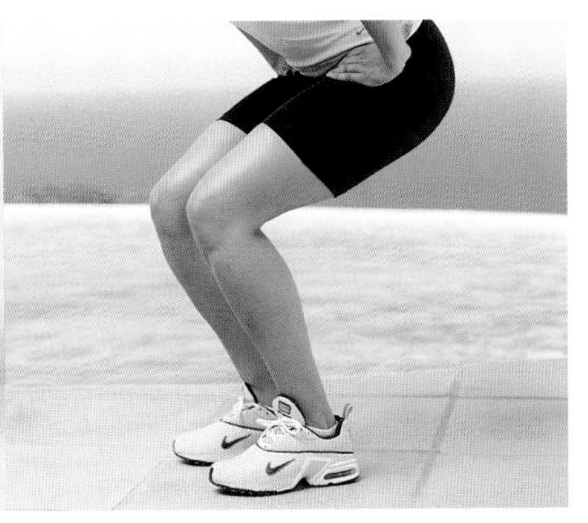

squat *p20*
① 25 reps ② 25 reps

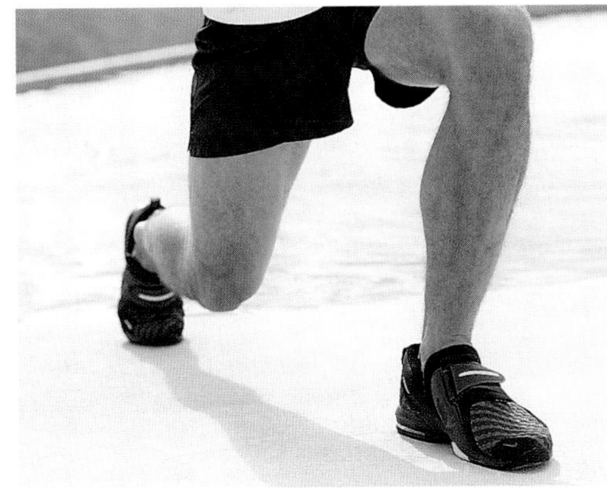

lunge *p56*
① 15 reps per leg ② 20 reps per leg

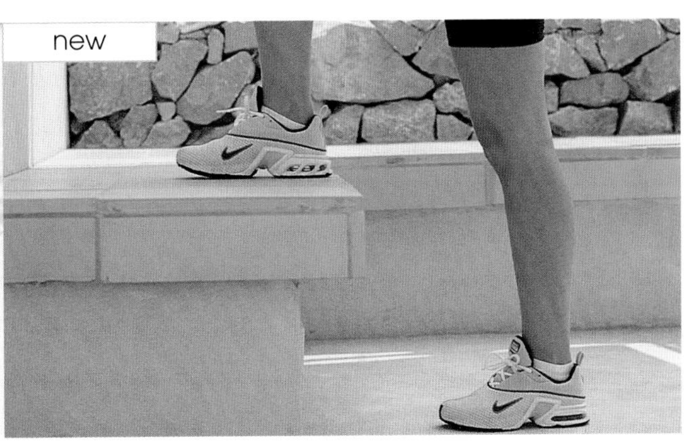

step-up *p62*
① 12 reps per leg ② 15 reps per leg x2

day 15 new exercises

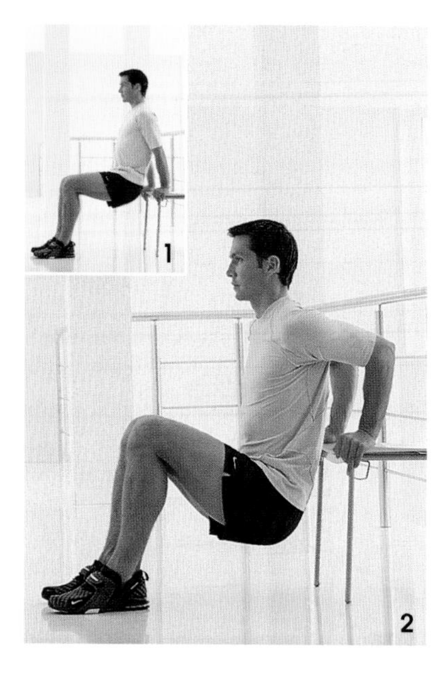

dip ◁

An intensive, effective exercise that challenges your upper body. Use a completely stable chair and place its back against a wall for safety.

1 Place your feet hip-width apart. Keeping your back straight and close to the front of the chair, bend your knees to 90°.

2 Lower yourself down until your arms are bent at 90°. Slowly push yourself back up until your arms are straight, but not locked.

upright row ▷

A great exercise for strength, tone, and stability in your shoulders and biceps.

1 Place your feet hip-width apart in the middle of the exertube. Keep your knees slightly bent and back straight. Cross the handles in front of you, palms facing your thighs.

2 Pull the handles up to chest height, leading with your elbows. Slowly lower your hands to the start position.

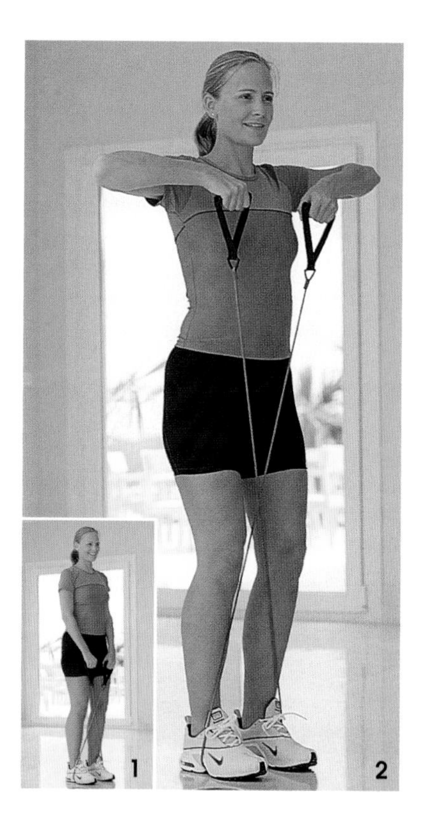

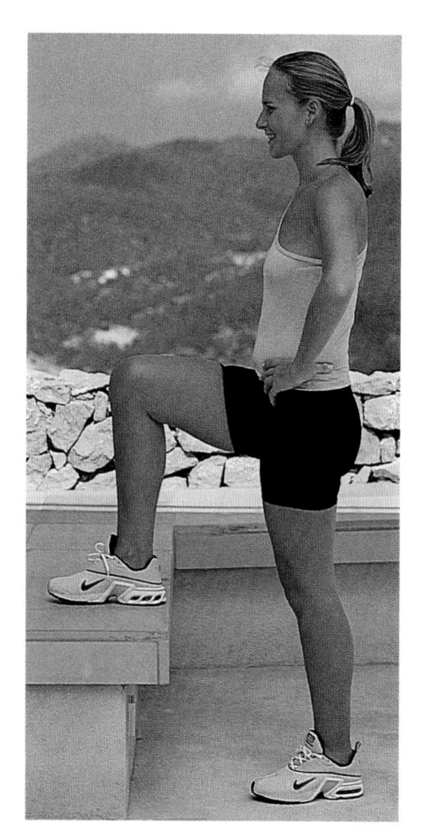

step-up ◁

This may look like a fairly basic exercise, but it's actually one of the most intensive for your lower body.

Stand facing a step or stair about 16 in (40 cm) high. Step up with one foot, placing your whole foot flat on the step. Keep your back straight and your head and neck relaxed, but in line with your torso. Step up with your other foot, so both feet are flat on the step. Step down with your leading foot first.

day 16

At some point during your rest day today, take a moment to settle yourself down somewhere quiet and comfortable to try a visualization exercise. It should help to harden your resolve to succeed.

In your mind's eye, imagine the body shape you'd like to have. Put your features on that body and memorize it. This is to be the new you. Then imagine yourself doing things that you never thought you could. This will be you once you've completed the plan – stronger, slimmer, more supple and active. Keep these two images in your mind – they're your reasons for succeeding.

eat&drink

breakfast wheat-free muesli *p132* **or** two slices of whole-wheat toast with nonhydrogenated spread and jam or jelly

lunch broccoli salad *p135* **or** Greek salad *p134*

dinner salmon and vegetable kabobs *p143* **or** steamed fish with salsa and salad *p144*

snacks banana, ½ oz (10 g) almonds, 2 oz (50 g) grapes **and** (for men) apple, and 4 oz (100 g) raspberries or 1 oz (25 g) raisins

drink at least 2½–3½ pints (1.5–2 liters) of water

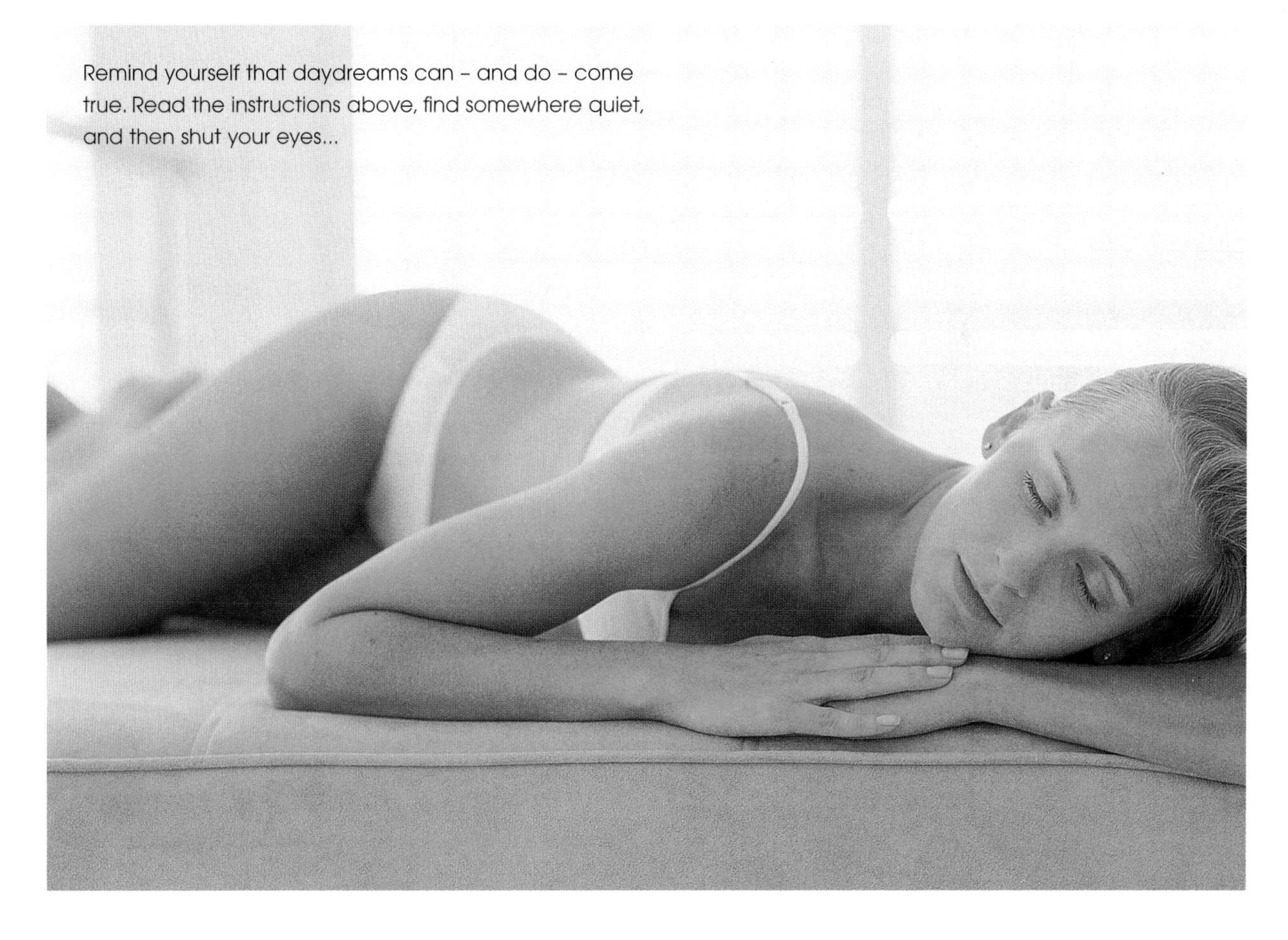

Remind yourself that daydreams can – and do – come true. Read the instructions above, find somewhere quiet, and then shut your eyes...

day 17

Today I'd like you to repeat the resistance work from day 15. Don't panic if your jeans felt tighter at the end of that session – or if it felt as though your muscles were growing. Sometimes when you work your body hard, it holds on to fluids in your muscles to help them recover. This is just a temporary thing. You're still getting leaner.

For variety, the cardio work for today is different from day 15. It's also shorter than your recent constant-pace sessions, but it is at a slightly higher intensity – 80% MHR (8/10 RPE). The interval training work you've done at a higher pace should help you sail through it.

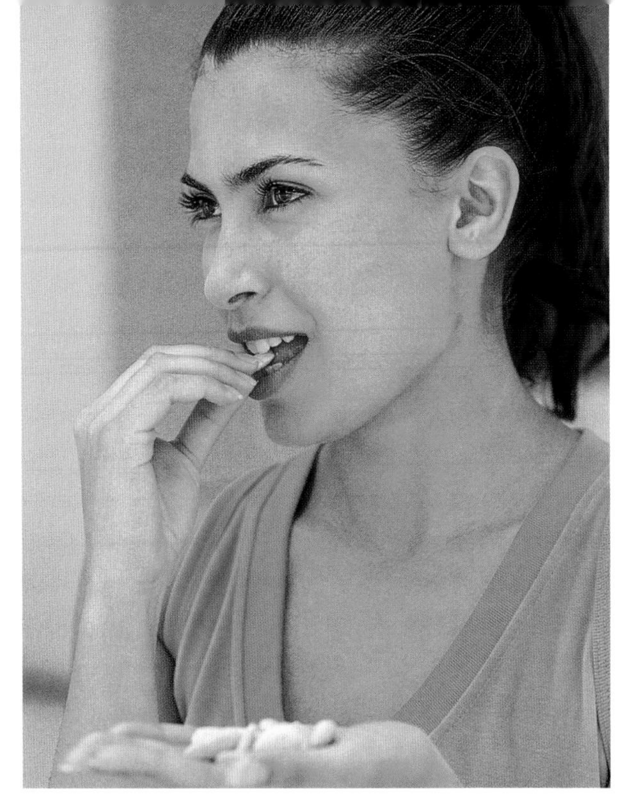

▽ Today's resistance is compound training – different exercises working the same muscle areas in different ways. The extended box push-up is one of those for upper arms.

△ After two weeks on the fat loss diet, you should have lost the cravings associated with high-sugar, high-fat foods. Strategic snacking can still ward off energy lows.

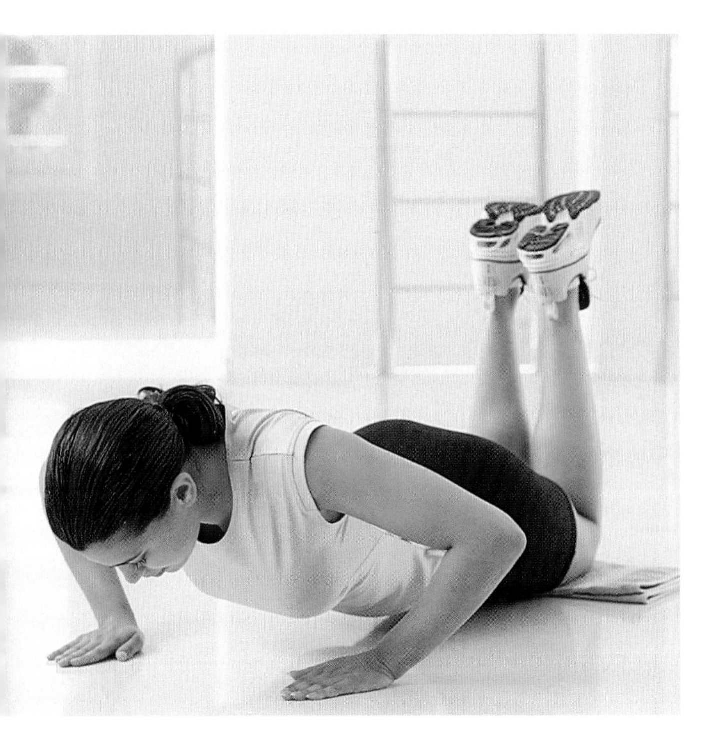

eat&drink

breakfast wheat-free muesli *p132* **or** oatmeal *p132*

lunch smoked salmon and dill salad *p138* **or** beet and carrot salad *p134*

dinner wheat-free pasta with turkey *p148* **or** steamed fish with Moroccan vegetables *p146*

snacks apple, pear, 1 oz (25 g) sunflower seeds, 1 oz (25 g) raisins **and** (for men) banana, 1 oz (25 g) sunflower seeds, ½ oz (10 g) raisins

drink at least 2½–3½ pints (1.5–2 liters) of water

three-part workout

Fast-pace walk or run at a constant pace for 30 minutes at 80% MHR (8/10 RPE), then repeat the resistance work from day 15. At the end of today's workout, finish with a short standing stretch (*p23*).

day 18

Both today and tomorrow are rest days, so you should feel as if you're having a mini-vacation. Even though you aren't going to be doing any exercise for the next 48 hours, keep your intake of water up. Count how many cups of coffee and tea you have over the course of the two days. They're diuretics, and my aim during the fat loss plan is to keep your body well-hydrated. Large amounts of coffee and tea will work against this.

If you find you're drinking more than two cups a day, aim to cut down. Substitute herbal teas or – better still – water. Do it gradually, though, since you might find your body suffers mild caffeine withdrawal symptoms, like headaches and lethargy.

eat & drink

breakfast whole-wheat pancakes *p132* **or** two slices of whole-wheat toast with nonhydrogenated spread and jam or jelly

lunch Camargue rice salad *p136* **or** wild rice salad *p136*

dinner smoked salmon and lentil salad *p147* **or** carrot and sweet potato fishcakes with herb salad *p144*

snacks apple, pear, and 4 oz (100 g) raspberries or 1 oz (25 g) dried apricots **and** (for men) 1 oz (25 g) mixed sunflower and sesame seeds, 1 oz (25 g) raisins

drink at least 2½–3½ pints (1.5–2 liters) of water

day 19

Two days off from exercising may not exactly be cause for celebration, but the chances are high that at some point during the eight-week fat loss plan you will want to go out for a meal. Far from being an unwelcome challenge, dinner in your favorite restaurant can be a treat – once you know what to ask for and what to avoid.

When you're ordering your food, steer clear of anything that's fried or deep-fried. Ask the waiter if it can be steamed, baked, or grilled instead. Creamy or buttery sauces are an absolute no-go area, too. Again, check with the waiter to see if your food can be cooked without them.

Don't pick at the contents of the bread basket. If the service is slow and you're feeling hungry, ask for some raw vegetables instead. And when you come to order your dessert, keep it simple and choose a fruit salad or Italian ice.

Of course, you may not be going out for dinner tonight. In which case, you have the choice of a mushroom risotto or a smoked salmon and lentil salad. Relish every mouthful and enjoy it!

eat & drink

breakfast fresh fruit salad with yogurt and seeds *p132* **or** oatmeal *p132*

lunch shrimp and linguine salad *p137* **or** wild rice salad *p136*

dinner mushroom risotto *p142* **or** smoked salmon and lentil salad *p147*

snacks banana, ½ oz (10 g) almonds, 2 oz (50 g) grapes **and** (for men) apple, and 4 oz (100 g) raspberries or 1 oz (25 g) raisins

drink at least 2½–3½ pints (1.5–2 liters) of water

day 20

After two days off, you'll either be looking forward to getting back to your exercise routine or feeling a little nervous about it. Either way, it's a good idea from time to time to check that you're doing all the exercises correctly. Sloppy work makes for a sloppy body. When you next have a few moments, look back through the plan for the step-by-steps for each exercise and make sure you're performing the movements as you should be.

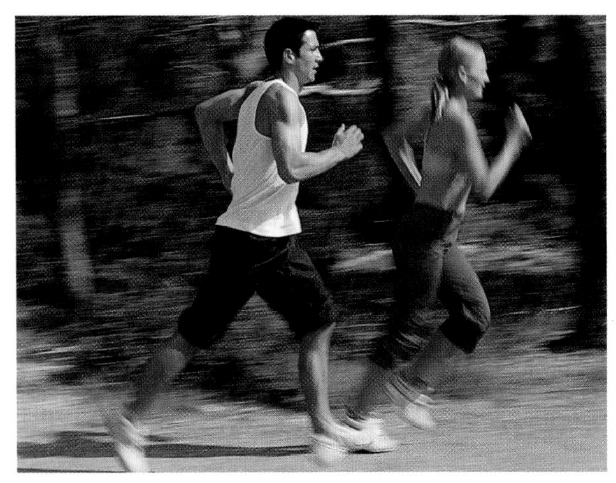

eat&drink

breakfast fresh fruit salad with yogurt and seeds *p132* **or** wheat-free muesli *p132*

lunch tuna sandwich *p138* **or** wild rice salad *p136*

dinner stuffed bell pepper *p142* **or** broiled fish with sweet potato and spinach bake *p144*

snacks apple, pear, 1 oz (25 g) sunflower seeds, 1 oz (25 g) raisins **and** (for men) banana, 1 oz (25 g) sunflower seeds, ½ oz (10 g) raisins

drink at least 2½–3½ pints (1.5–2 liters) of water

three-part workout

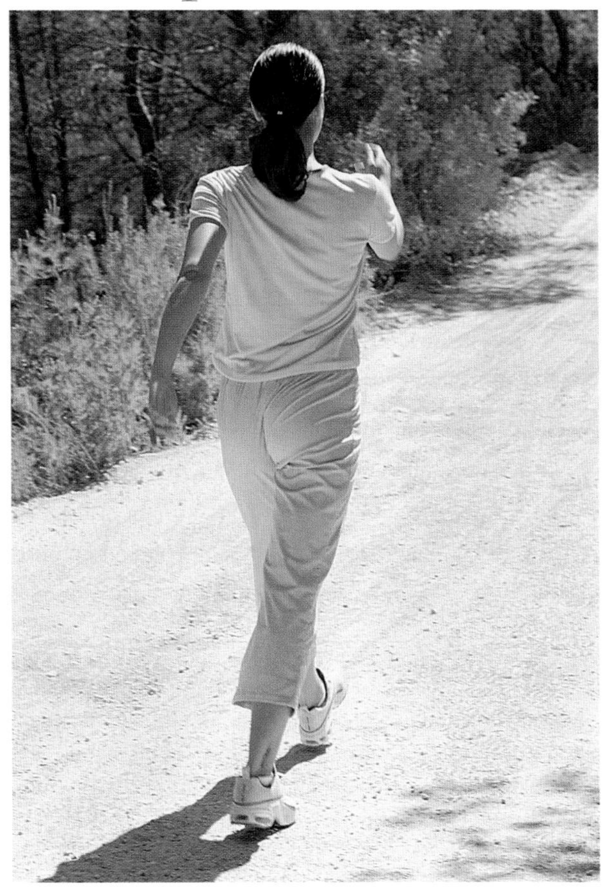

1 cardio

In the interval training today, run at 85% MHR (8–9/10 RPE). Start by fast-pace walking for 1 minute, then run for 1 minute. Repeat 11 times, so you walk and run 12 times.

2 resistance

The training for today falls into two groups. Do the reps for the first four exercises in order, rest for 2 minutes, then repeat. Rest again for 2 minutes, then do the reps for the other seven exercises in order. Rest, then repeat them.

3 stretching

Finish the workout with a total body stretch (*p22*).

day 20 resistance work

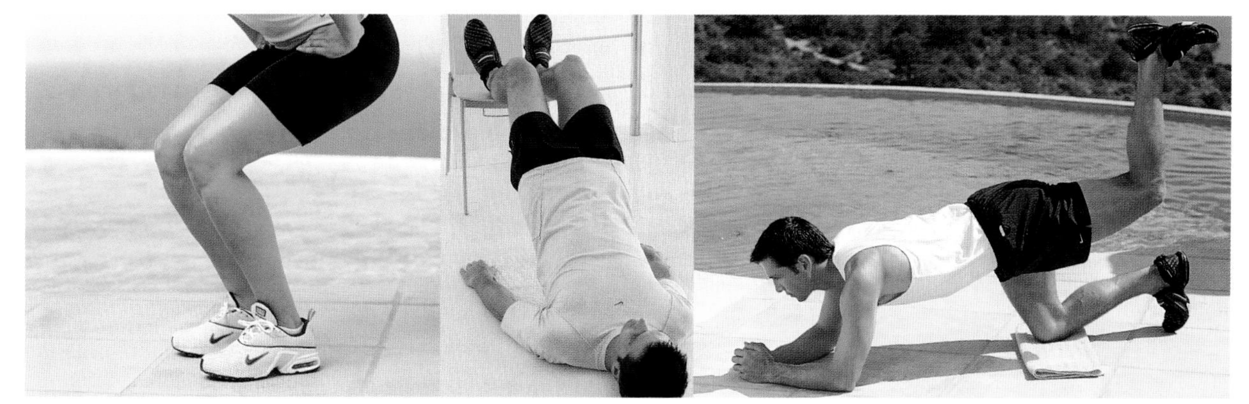

squat *p20*
① 12 reps ② 20 reps

body raise *p20*
① 12 reps ② 20 reps

glute raise *p38*
① 12 reps per leg ② 20 reps per leg

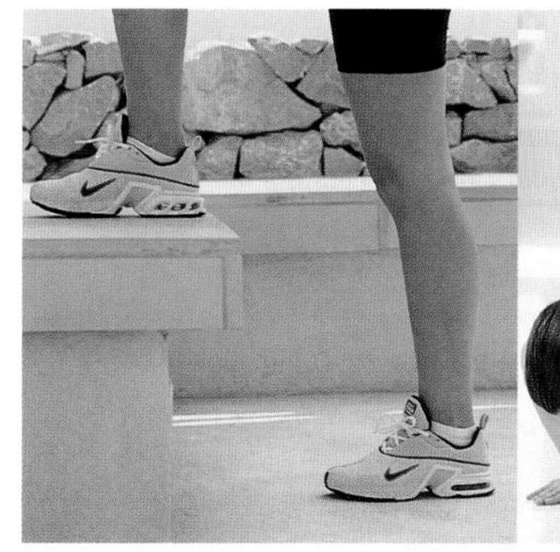

step-up *p62*
① 12 per leg ② 15 per leg x2

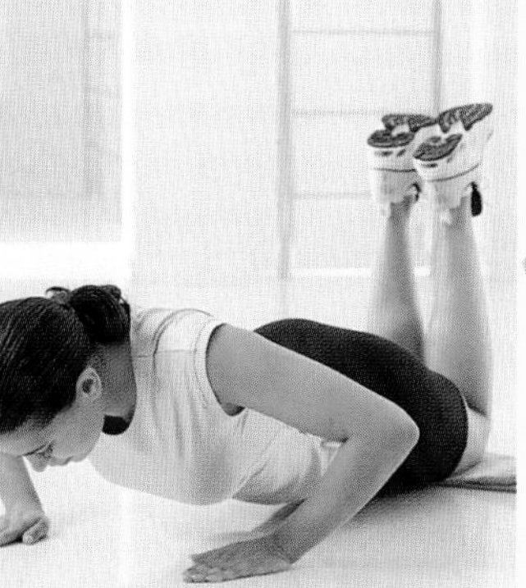

extended box push-up *p56*
① 20 reps ② 30 reps

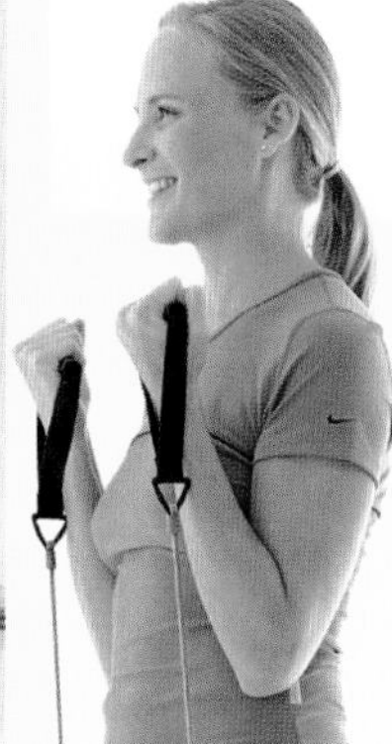

bicep curl *p21*
① 15 reps ② 20 reps

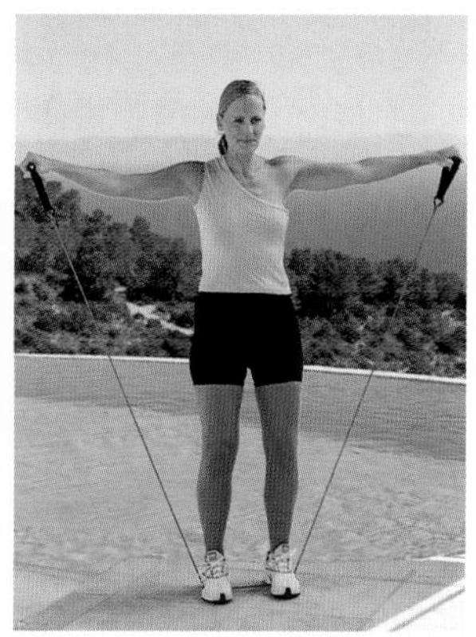

lateral raise *p21*
① 15 reps ② 20 reps

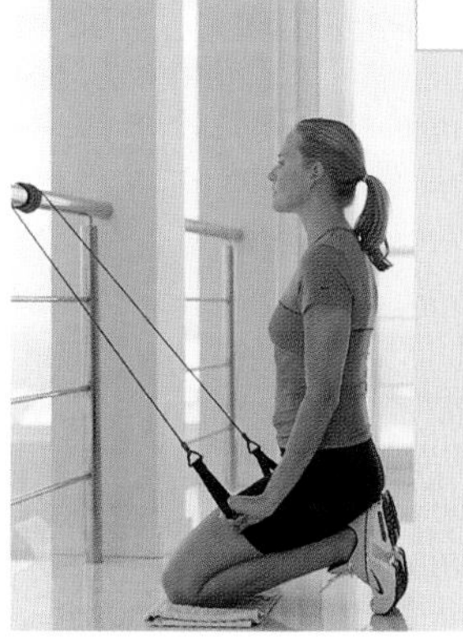

tricep press *p56*
① 12 reps ② 15 reps

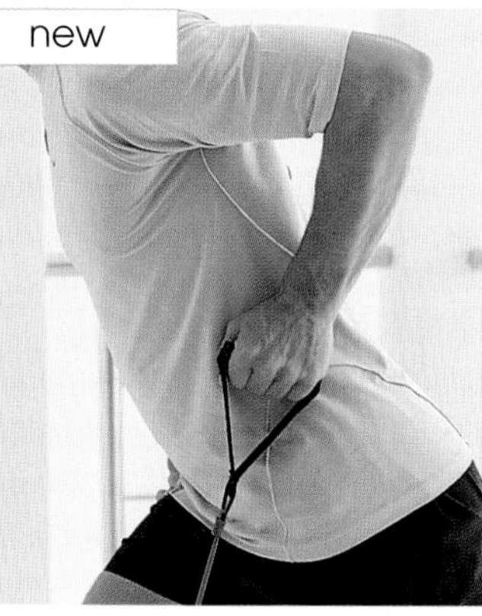

single arm row *p68*
① & ② 15 reps per arm

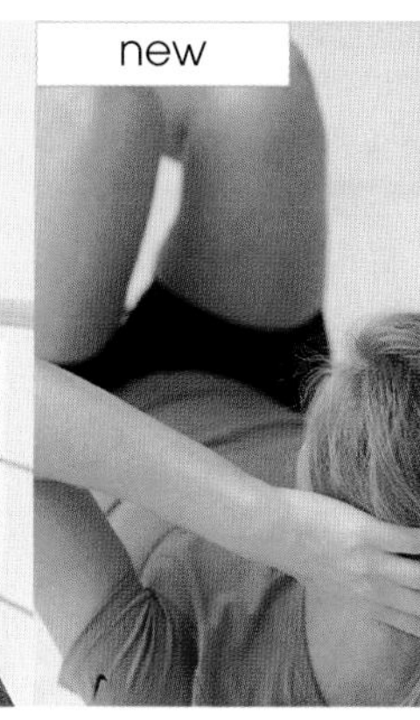

full crunch *p68*
①15 reps ② 20 reps

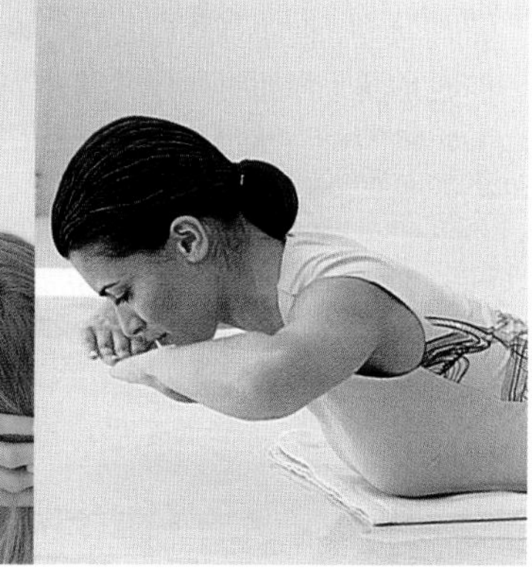

back extension *p38*
① 15 reps ② 20 reps x2

day 20 new exercises

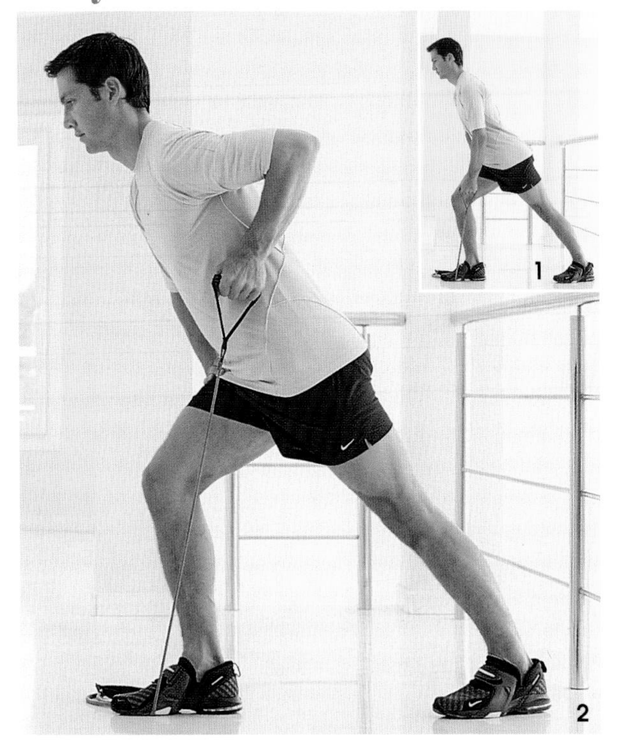

single-arm row ◁

Focus on pulling your shoulder blades together as you do the exercise and you'll soon have a good excuse for showing off your back.

1 Place one foot about one-third of the way along the exertube. Place your other foot about one stride-length behind you. Hold the handle of the short end with one hand, arm relaxed, and place your other hand on your thigh. Keeping your hips facing straight ahead, bring your body forward. Aim to keep your head and body at 45° and make sure your front knee stays above your toes.

2 Pull the handle of the exertube up toward your chest, until your elbow is at right angles close to your body. Keep your body stable, your back straight, and your shoulders relaxed. Slowly return to the start position.

full crunch ▷

A combination of the crunch and the reverse curl, the full crunch works the whole of your tummy area.

1 Lie on your back with your legs in the air, your knees bent, and your legs together. Place your hands behind your head.

2 Breathe out, curling your legs and pelvis toward your rib cage as you do so. At the same time, curl your shoulders forward. Take care not to tense the muscles of your neck. Slowly return to the start position, breathing out at the same time.

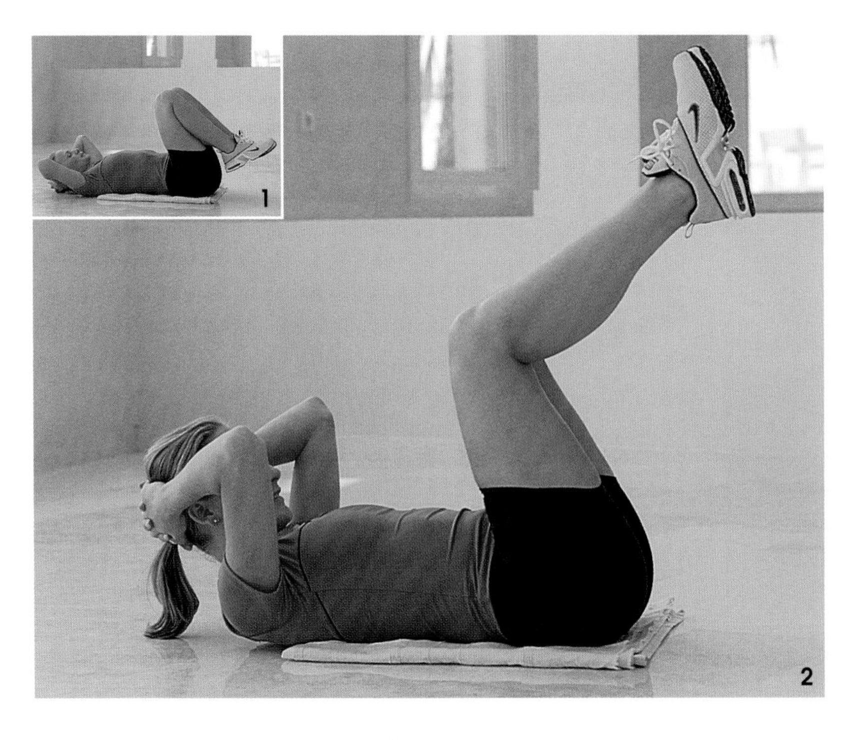

day 21

You've already had a 'cardio only' day, but this is your first 'resistance only' day. The session is a repeat of the resistance work from day 20 and is relatively tough because it covers a lot of muscle areas and you have to do a lot of reps.

▷ A smoothie is a simple and delicious start to the day. For those who really can't face eating too much for breakfast, it has particular appeal.

▽ Exercising with a friend or partner takes some of the pain away. What's more, you'll have someone to encourage you when you're feeling loath to work out.

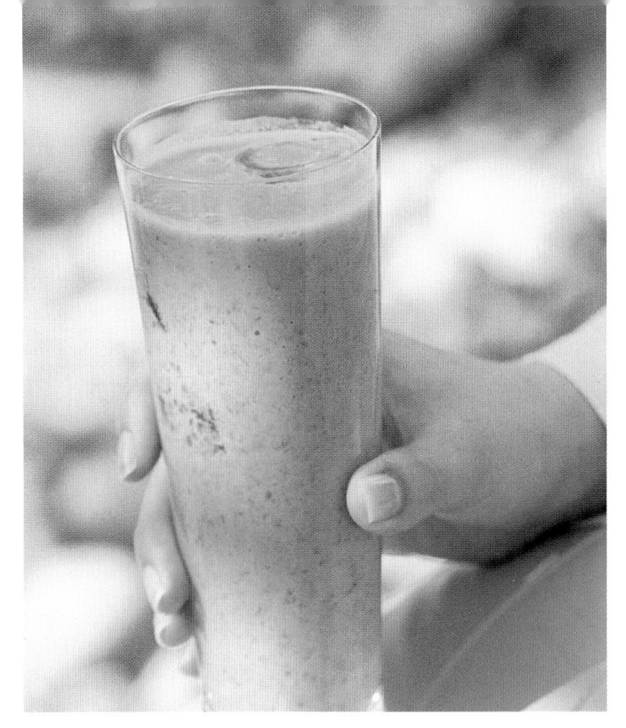

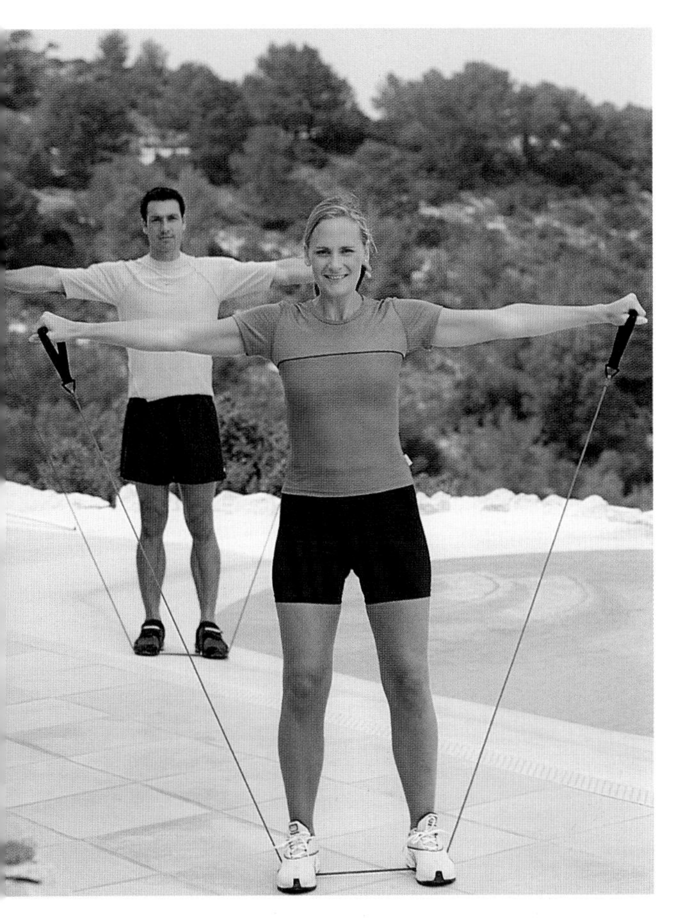

eat&drink

breakfast two slices of whole-wheat toast with nonhydrogenated spread and jam or jelly **or** wheat-free muesli *p132*

lunch broccoli salad *p135* **or** Greek salad *p134*

dinner salmon and vegetable kabobs *p143* **or** steamed fish with salsa and salad *p144*

snacks apple, pear, and 4 oz (100 g) raspberries or 1 oz (25 g) dried apricots **and** (for men) 1 oz (25 g) mixed sunflower and sesame seeds, 1 oz (25 g) raisins

drink at least 2½–3½ pints (1.5–2 liters) of water

two-part workout

This is a 'resistance only' day, so there's no cardio training to do. Focus your mind on the resistance work. This is a repeat of the compound training exercises from day 20 and it will probably be quite testing for you. At the end of the session, make sure you ward off any stiffness or soreness in your muscles by taking your time to do a total body stretch (*p22*).

week 4

You're getting **into the routine** now. Make it through this week and you're **halfway** there. In a sense, you've come through the hardest part: you've discovered **your health**. All we have to do now is make it work fully for you. When one of my better-known **clients** was asked recently why she trained with me, her response was, 'He gets results. He's my personal motivation.' **Let me be yours.**

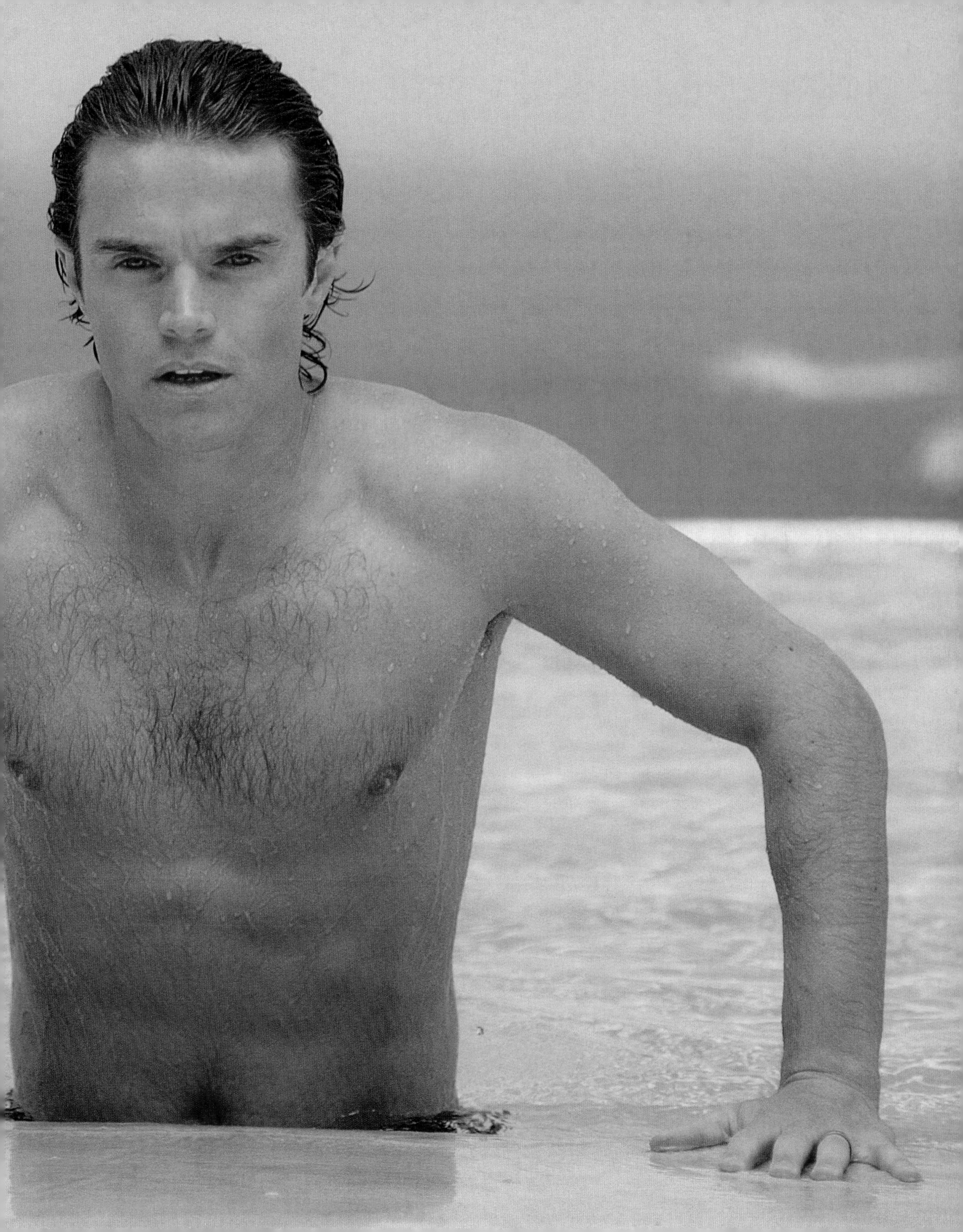

day 22

On your rest day today, take some time to bring your calendar up to date. Make sure you know which are your exercise days over the coming weeks, then check that work commitments and social engagements aren't getting in the way.

Write down your new personal goals, and revisit those you've been jotting down since you started the plan. If any of them have slipped, put them in your calendar again. It doesn't matter too much what they are – you could be aiming to work harder during your cardio sessions, or trying to cut out coffee or tea. Writing them down will help.

Now read the notes you've made on the workouts themselves, and your feelings about them just after you'd done them. Going through these, you might be pleasantly surprised by how much progress you've made in just 21 days.

eat&drink

breakfast fresh fruit salad with yogurt and seeds *p132* **or** wheat-free muesli *p132*

lunch tuna sandwich *p138* **or** wild rice salad *p136*

dinner stuffed bell pepper *p142* **or** broiled fish with sweet potato and spinach bake *p144*

snacks banana, ½ oz (10 g) almonds, 2 oz (50 g) grapes **and** (for men) apple, and 4 oz (100 g) raspberries or 1 oz (25 g) raisins

drink at least 2½–3½ pints (1.5–2 liters) of water

▷ Make a record in your calendar of your new personal goals for the week. Remember, be realistic about what is and isn't possible. Poor goal-setting will only lead to disappointment and feelings of failure on your part.

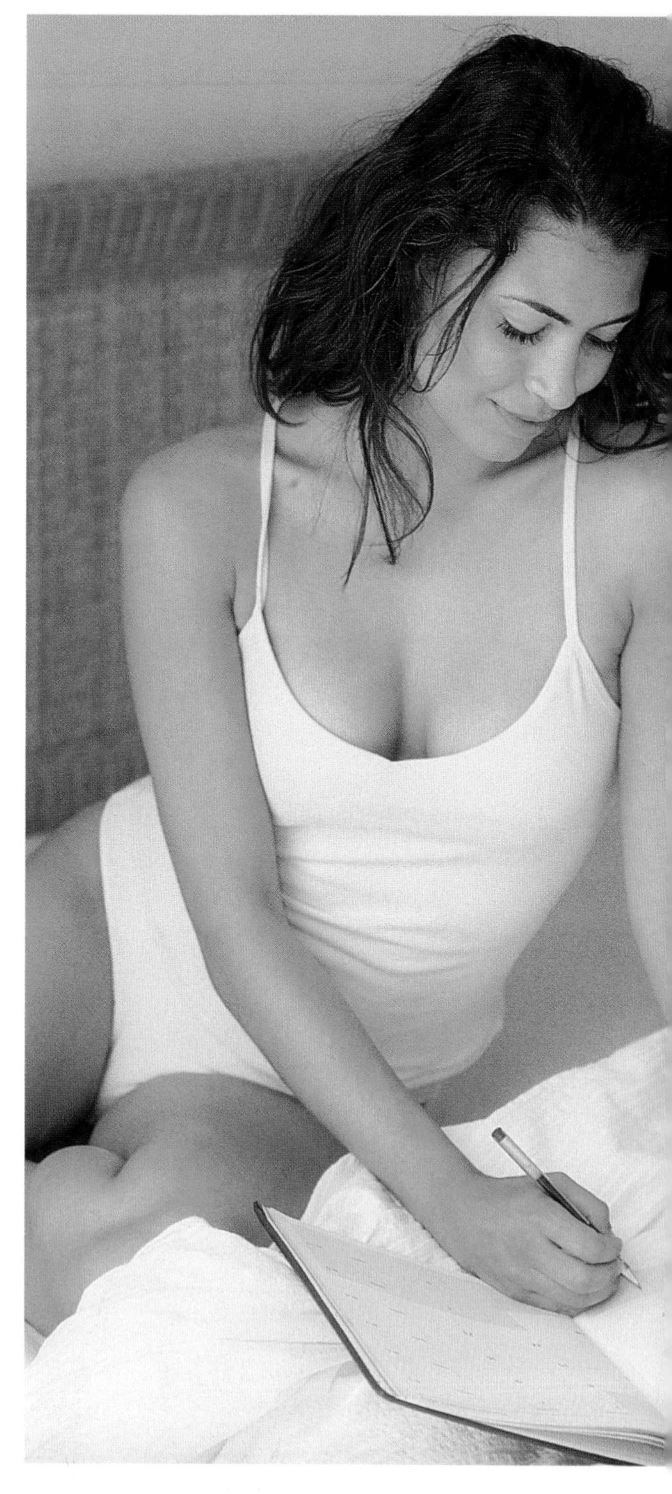

day 23

One of the most effective things I do for myself in terms of exercise is add variety. Just when I'm getting used to one type of cardio training, I change it, or add something new. By doing this, I'm working my body in a totally different way. I'm forcing it to adapt to change. It's then that it burns the most calories.

So, instead of running or fast-pace walking this week, try some other kind of cardio training – swimming or cycling, perhaps. The change will do you good both physically and psychologically. You should be fairly used to using the RPE scale by now, so you'll be able to gauge whether you're working at the correct level. Just make sure your sessions are the same length of time as those I recommend. And move on to the resistance part of the workout as quickly as you can.

eat&drink

breakfast poached egg on two slices of dry whole-wheat toast **or** vegetable omelet *p133*

lunch Greek salad *p134* **or** quinoa salad *p136*

dinner marinated tuna with polenta *p145* **or** chicken with couscous and mint yogurt *p149*

snacks apple, pear, 1 oz (25 g) sunflower seeds, 1 oz (25 g) raisins **and** (for men) banana, 1 oz (25 g) sunflower seeds, ½ oz (10 g) raisins

drink at least 2½–3½ pints (1.5–2 liters) of water

three-part workout

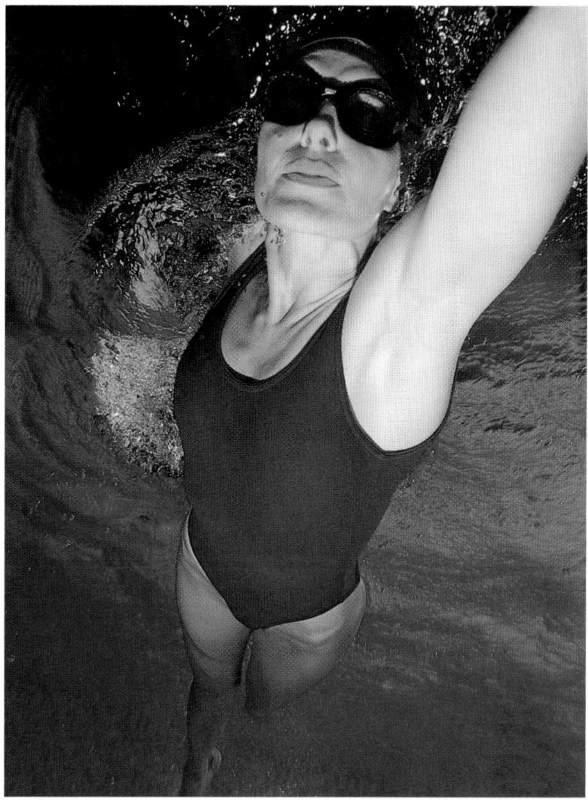

1 cardio

Run or fast-pace walk at a constant pace for 40 minutes. Work at 70–75% MHR (7/10 RPE). If you prefer, you can swim or cycle for the same amount of time, as long as you do it at the same level of intensity.

2 resistance

Your resistance program today is based on PHA training. Perform the reps for the exercises in order, with 10-second rests in between them, then repeat them all (with rests). Level ② users, make sure you have plenty of resistance on your exertube (*see day 9*).

3 stretching

Round off today's session with a total body stretch (*p22*).

day 23 resistance work

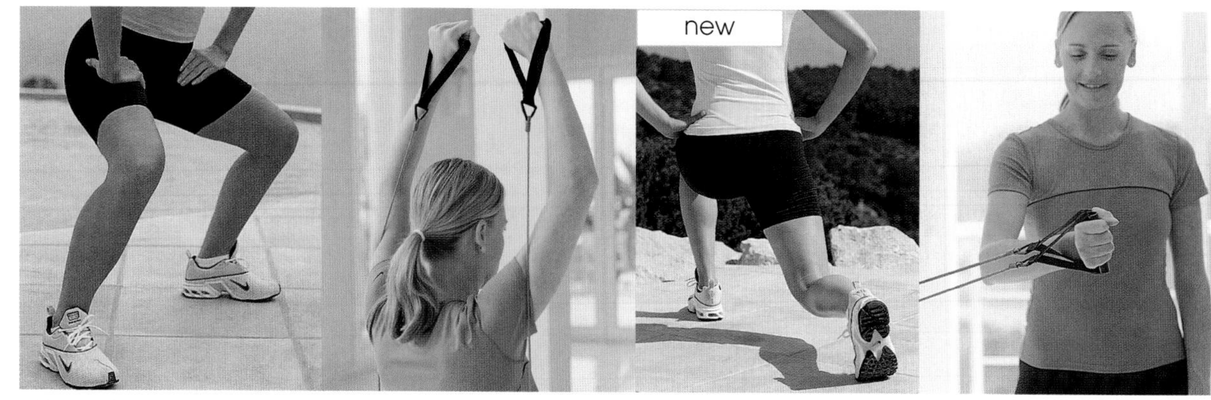

wide squat *p52*
① 20 reps ② 25 reps

shoulder press *p52*
① 25 reps ② 15 reps

walking lunge *p75*
① 20 strides ② 20 strides

pec fly *p52*
① 20 per arm ② 15 per arm

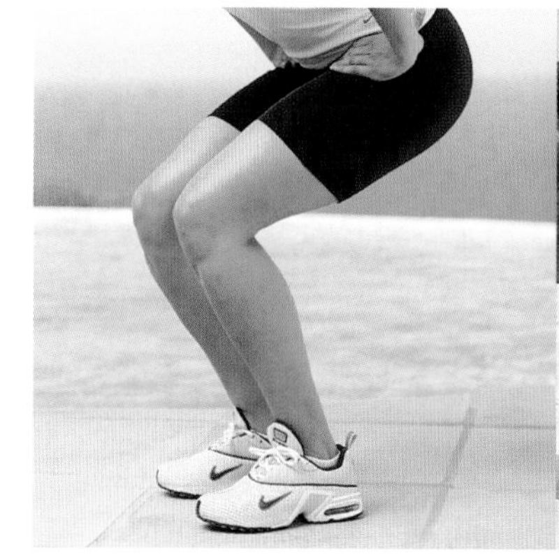

squat *p20*
① 20 reps ② 25 reps

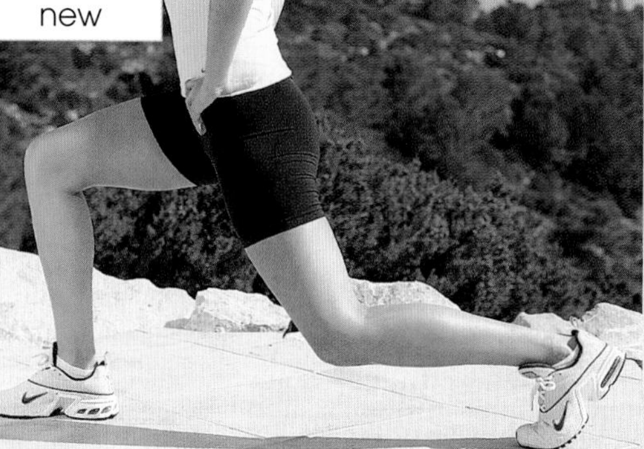

power lunge *p75*
① 15 reps per leg ② 15 reps per leg

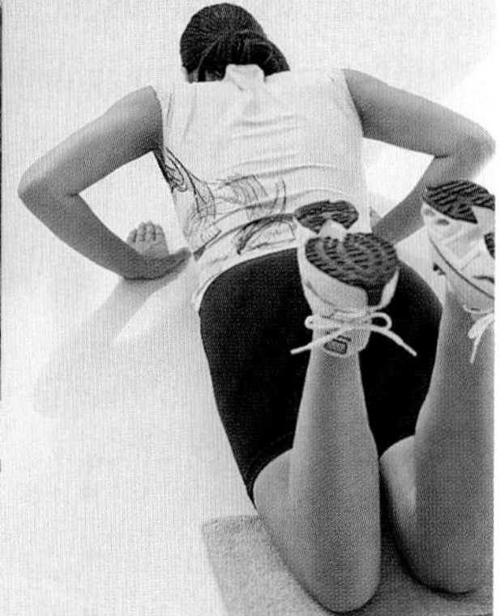

extended box push-up *p56*
① 20 reps ② 25 reps

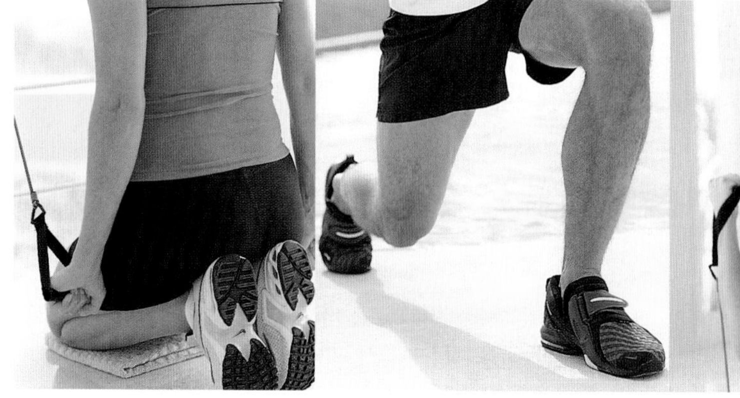

tricep press *p56*
① 15 reps ② 15 reps

lunge *p56*
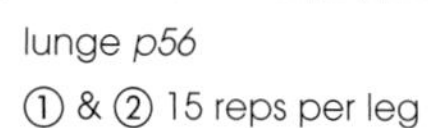
① & ② 15 reps per leg

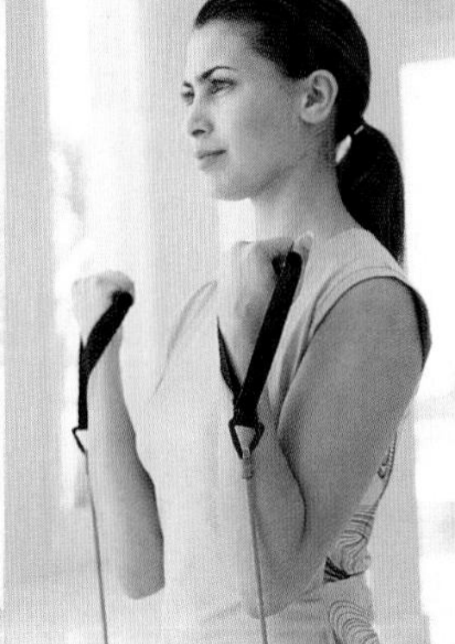

bicep curl *p21*
① 15 reps ② 12 reps

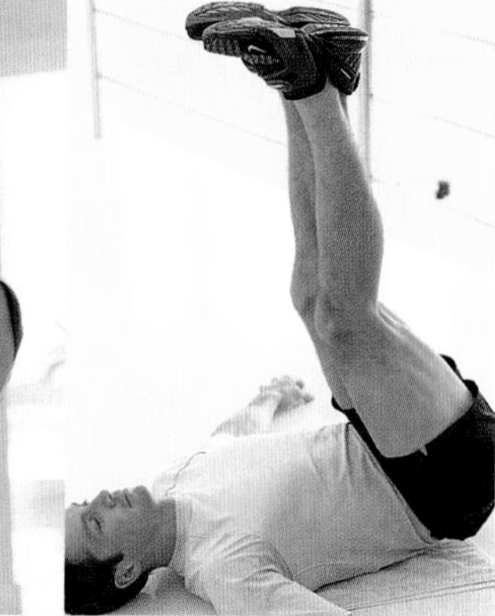

reverse curl *p43*
① & ② 25 reps x2

day 23 new exercises

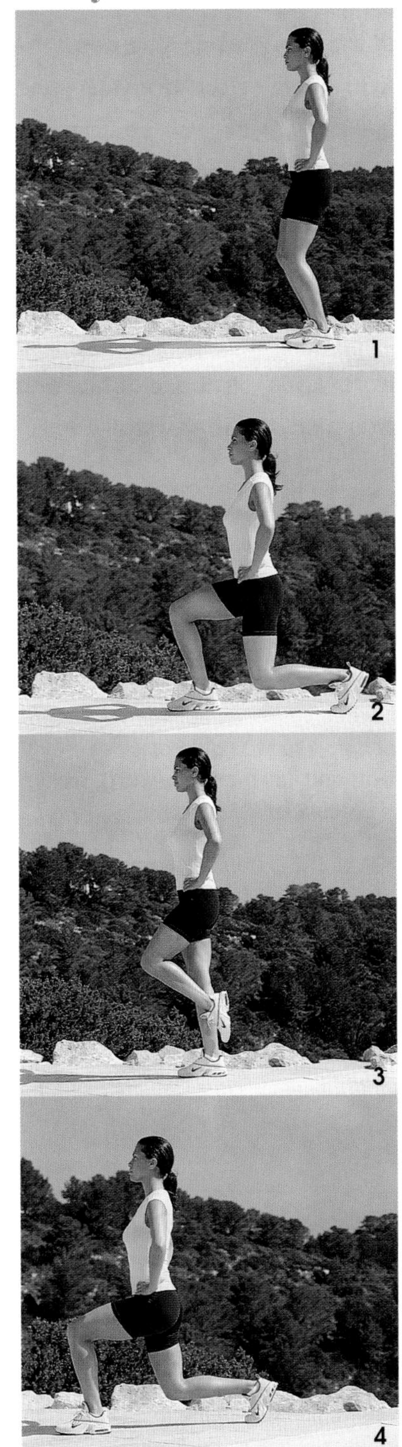

walking lunge ◁

To begin with, you may find it hard to balance while you do the walking lunge, but persevere – once you've perfected the technique, it will give you stronger legs that look longer. Clear yourself some space so you can take two or three strides one after the other.

1 Stand with your feet hip-width apart, knees slightly bent. Rest your hands on your hips. Keep your back staight and your tummy muscles pulled in.

2 Step forward so that your front foot is about one stride-length from your back foot. Lower your body as you do this, then hold the position for 1 second.

3 Raise your body, then step forward with the other leg to repeat the lunge.

4 Lower your body as you did in step 2, then continue from step 3.

power lunge ▷

This is a more difficult, more explosive version of the 'basic' lunge. It really gets to work on your leg muscles and raises your heart rate. Keep the movement steady and controlled.

1 Stand with your feet hip-width apart and your hands on your hips.

2 Take a step forward so that your front foot is about one stride-length from your back foot. As you step forward, lower your body. Make sure your front knee doesn't move beyond your toes. Spring back to the start position, pushing through with the heel of your front foot as you do so. Try not to let your body waver.

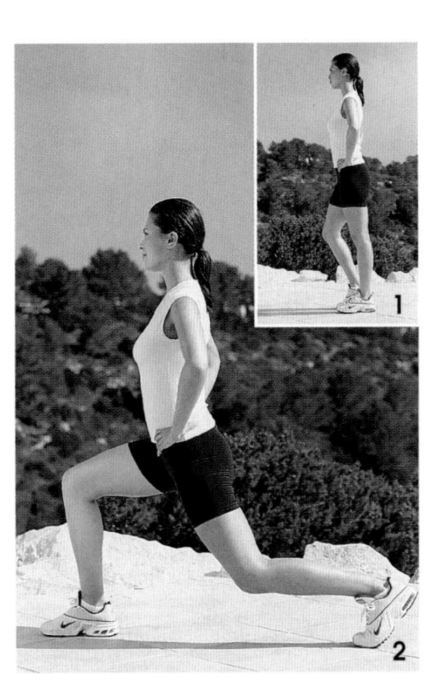

day 24

Never underestimate your body's need for nutrients at lunchtime on your rest days. You may not be working out, but you still need energy to sustain you through the afternoon. And if you skip lunch, you risk having an energy dip that could tempt you to snack on something sweet.

The way I've arranged the fat loss diet, you start every day with a wholesome breakfast to boost energy levels when they're at their lowest. This is your most important meal and you should never miss it.

In the middle of the day – when you need the most energy – you have your heaviest and starchiest meal. Generally, it consists of complex carbohydrates, which will fuel your body through the afternoon. And in the evening – when you need less energy because you'll be resting through the night – your dinner is light and easy to digest. Usually, it's a combination of vegetables and protein. Remember to keep off the alcohol and instead enjoy it with a glass of mineral water.

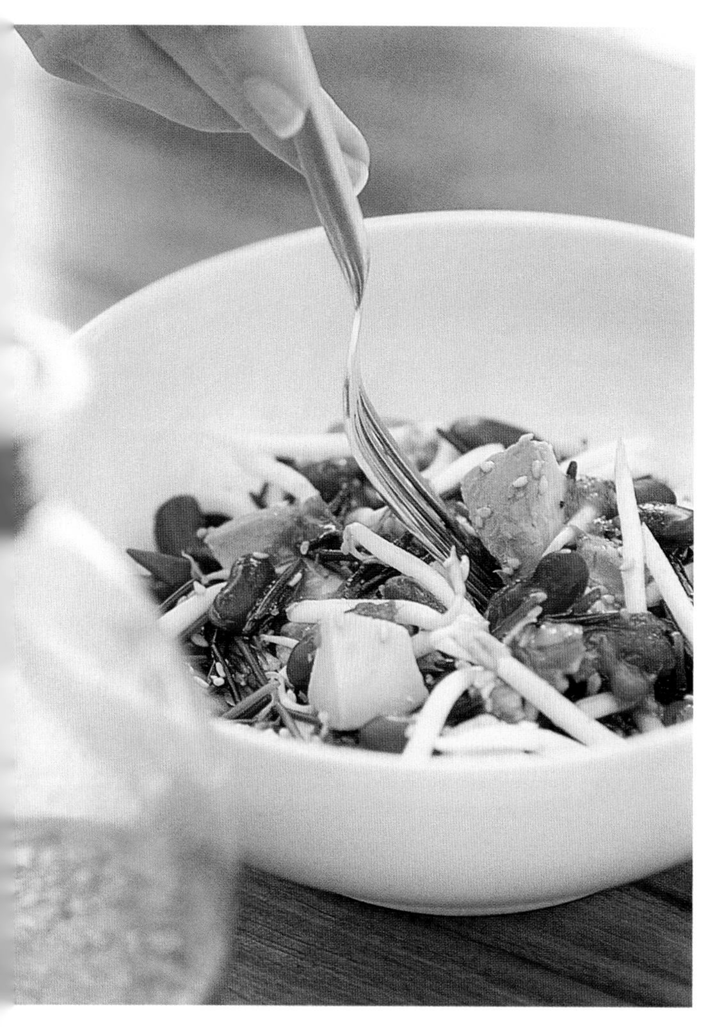

eat&drink

breakfast wheat-free muesli *p132* **or** oatmeal *p132*

lunch wild rice salad *p136* **or** Camargue rice salad *p136*

dinner steamed fish with Moroccan vegetables *p146* **or** broiled fish with sweet potato and spinach bake *p144*

snacks apple, pear, and 4 oz (100 g) raspberries or 1 oz (25 g) dried apricots **and** (for men) 1 oz (25 g) mixed sunflower and sesame seeds, 1 oz (25 g) raisins

drink at least 2½–3½ pints (1.5–2 liters) of water

◁ Never be tempted to skip lunch. A meal like this wild rice salad (*p136*) has the perfect mix of vegetables and complex carbohydrates to give you all the energy you need for the afternoon.

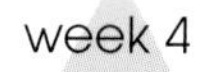

day 25

This is another 'cardio only' day and it's a tough one because it's a 45-minute session. To prevent tiredness – and the injuries that could arise from that – pay close attention to your technique.

eat&drink

breakfast fresh fruit salad with yogurt and seeds *p132* **or** oatmeal *p132*

lunch shrimp and linguine salad *p137* **or** beet and carrot salad *p134*

dinner sweet potato gnocchi with tomato and shrimp sauce *p140* **or** broiled or steamed fish with quinoa *p143*

snacks banana, ½ oz (10 g) almonds, 2 oz (50 g) grapes **and** (for men) apple, and 4 oz (100 g) raspberries or 1 oz (25 g) raisins

drink at least 2½–3½ pints (1.5–2 liters) of water

two-part workout

Instead of running or fast-pace walking, you can swim or cycle, if you prefer. Make sure you work at the same level of intensity and for the same length of time.

1 cardio

Run or fast-pace walk at a constant pace for 45 minutes. Work at 70–75% MHR (7–8/10 RPE).

2 stretching

Finish off today's two-part workout by performing a short standing stretch (*p23*).

the best running technique

Running is a high-intensity, high-impact exercise that requires more power than fast-pace walking. Good technique is everything. Here are my top 10 tips:

- Get a pair of good running shoes to cushion and support your feet and ankles. Because running is a high-impact exercise, those with knee problems should not attempt it.
- It may sound odd, but don't try too hard. Running with

▽ Short strides are better than long ones. Keep your feet close to the ground and land on your heels, then roll through your whole foot. Swinging your arms forward and backward (inset) helps your momentum.

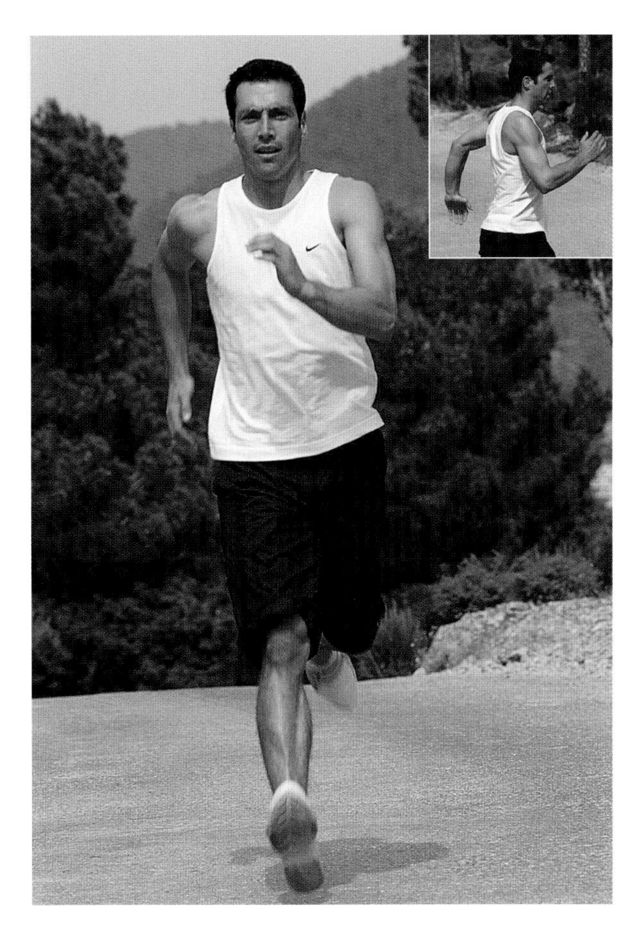

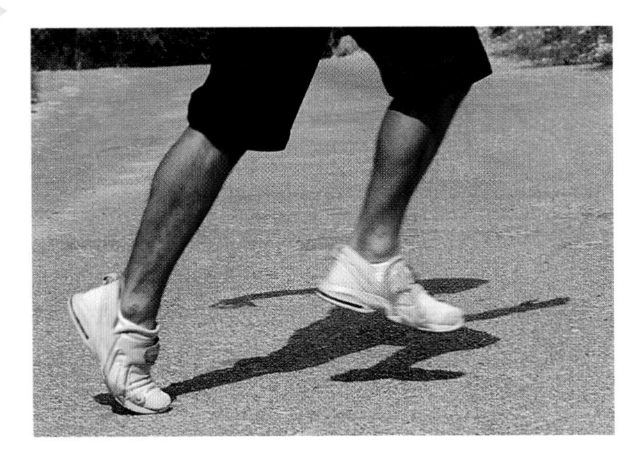

△ Take off from your toes, using the muscles of your bottom and the backs of your thighs to power you. You should be able to feel your buttock muscles working – if you can't, look again at your technique.

high knee-lifts, long strides, and big, bouncy steps will only tire you out and put strain on your joints.

- Short, fast strides are better than long ones.
- Keep your neck extended and your shoulders down in a relaxed, comfortable position. Every so often during your run, check your shoulders and pull them down, if necessary.
- Use your arms to help your momentum. Swing them forward and backward, but don't exaggerate the action. And relax your hands – don't tense them into fists.
- Keep your body upright and straight, and your tummy muscles pulled in.
- Make sure you use the muscles of your bottom to push power through your legs and propel you forward.
- Keep your feet close to the ground.
- Land on your heels, then roll through the whole foot.
- Take off from your toes.

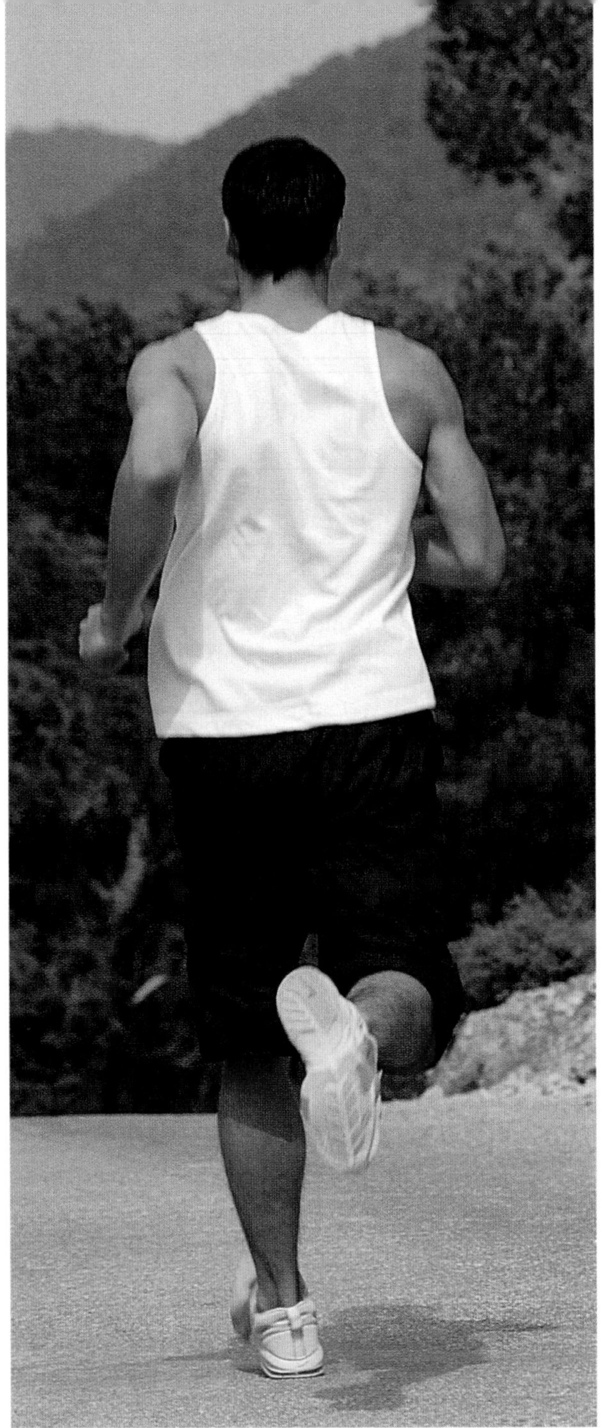

△ Keep your shoulders in a relaxed, comfortable position. As you run, check them from time to time and pull them down if you find you've been pulling them up. And keep your back straight – this helps to diffuse tension in your upper body.

day 26

After the tough cardio session yesterday, take a few moments to do some extra stretching today. Not only will this reduce any muscle soreness and stiffness, it will leave you with longer, leaner, and more flexible muscles, too.

Getting into the habit of stretching every day is a good idea, anyway. And the older you get, the more important it becomes to maintain your flexibility. Spend about 10 minutes every day performing the total body stretch. In place of the last two stretch moves (as they are on page 22), perform the hamstring stretch (lying down) and the quadricep stretch (lying down).

eat&drink

breakfast whole-wheat pancakes *p132* **or** fresh fruit salad with yogurt and seeds *p132*

lunch asparagus and artichoke salad *p135* **or** smoked salmon and dill salad *p138*

dinner polenta-crusted swordfish with sweet potato *p146* **or** lemon shrimp with three bean salad *p148*

snacks apple, pear, 1 oz (25 g) sunflower seeds, 1 oz (25 g) raisins **and** (for men) banana, 1 oz (25 g) sunflower seeds, ½ oz (10 g) raisins

drink at least 2½–3½ pints (1.5–2 liters) of water

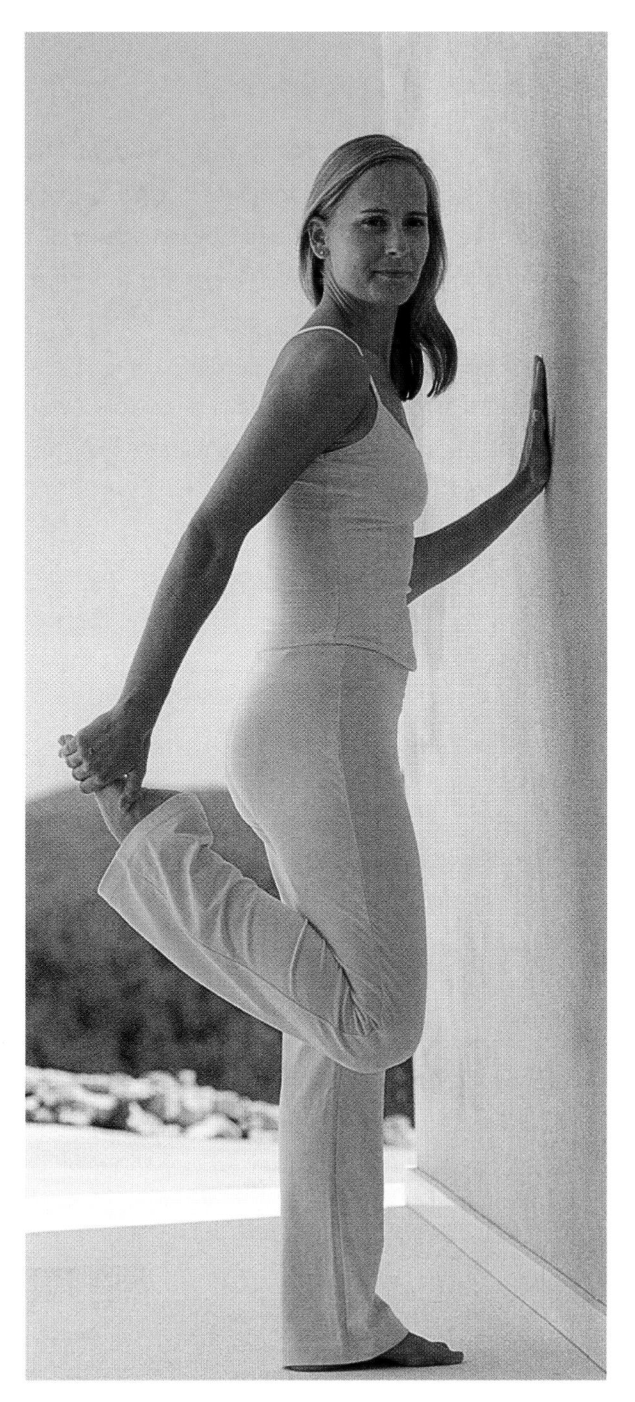

△ The quadricep stretch (*p26*) is great for easing soreness and stiffness in the muscles of your thighs. If you find yourself becoming a little wobbly as you're doing it, you may want to support yourself by standing against a wall or rail.

Stretching may seem a bit boring, but your improved **flexibility** makes it all worthwhile.

day 27

As you approach the halfway mark, you will be feeling quite different from four weeks ago, and it's workouts like today's that have helped you make the progress. If you think you're getting too tired, however, make sure you're working within your optimum training zone (*p17*).

The resistance work for today is a repeat of day 23, but I've changed the cardio to interval training.

eat&drink

breakfast two slices of whole-wheat toast with nonhydrogenated spread and jam or jelly **or** wheat-free muesli *p132*

lunch broccoli salad *p135* **or** Greek salad *p134*

dinner salmon and vegetable kabobs *p143* **or** vegetable and tofu kabobs *p142*

snacks apple, pear, and 4 oz (100 g) raspberries or 1 oz (25 g) dried apricots **and** (for men) 1 oz (25 g) mixed sunflower and sesame seeds, 1 oz (25 g) raisins

drink at least 2½–3½ pints (1.5–2 liters) of water

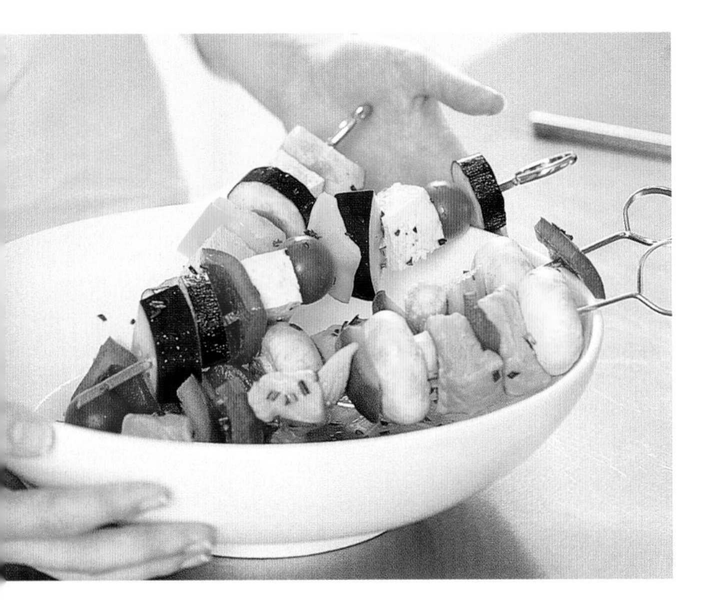

three-part workout

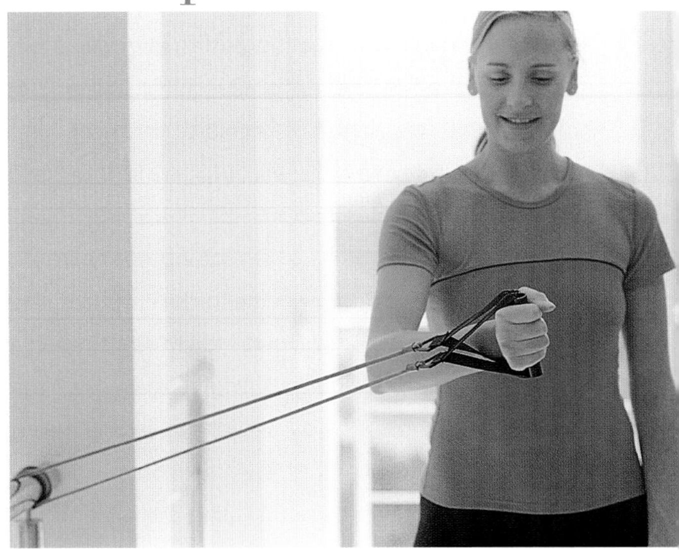

1 cardio

Fast-pace walk for 3 minutes, then run for 2 minutes. Repeat seven times so that you walk and run a total of eight times each. Run at 85% MHR (8–9/10 RPE). These are quite long intervals performed at a high level, so make sure you're breathing deeply.

2 resistance

Repeat the resistance work from day 23. Remember to perform the reps for the exercises in order, with 10-second rests in between them. Then repeat the sequence.

3 stretching

Round off today's workout by performing a total body sequence (*p22*).

◁ Marinating is a simple but effective way to intensify flavors. You can prepare these kabobs (*p143–144*) up to 24 hours ahead of time and then pop them in the fridge: they'll be even tastier as a result.

day 28

Another 'cardio only' day. This is a 45-minute session, so make sure you keep yourself well-hydrated throughout it. This is equally important when you're doing your resistance work, by the way. Many people tend to think they need less then, because they aren't sweating as much. But resistance work depletes a large amount of water from your muscles, and a process called acidic buildup starts to take place. It's this that's responsible for making your muscles feel sore and stiff. So drink plenty.

eat&drink

breakfast wheat-free muesli *p132* **or** oatmeal *p132*

lunch smoked salmon sandwich *p139* **or** wild rice salad *p136*

dinner broiled or steamed fish with quinoa *p143* **or** steamed fish with salsa and salad *p144*

snacks banana, ½ oz (10 g) almonds, 2 oz (50 g) grapes **and** (for men) apple, and 4 oz (100 g) raspberries or 1 oz (25 g) raisins

drink at least 2½–3½ pints (1.5–2 liters) of water

If you **demand a lot** from yourself at this stage, you can be sure **you'll attain it.**

two-part workout

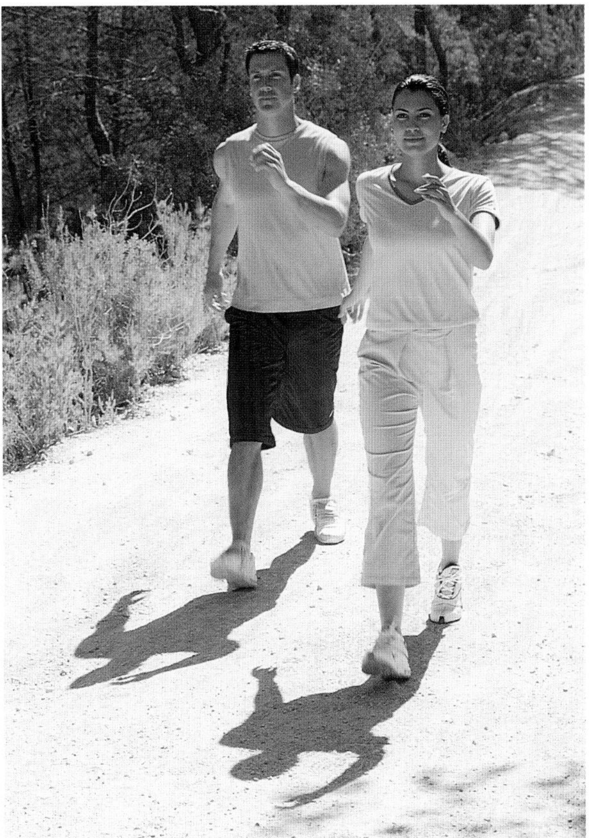

1 cardio

Run or fast-pace walk at a constant pace for 45 minutes. Work at 75% MHR (7–8/10 RPE). Although this session is quite long, the intensity is relatively low. As you do it, think back to how you felt when you were doing the sessions during your first week. Is your breathing any easier now? Has your technique improved? Compare yourself now with then. You may be pleasantly surprised.

2 stretching

At the end of today's cardio workout, perform a short standing stretch (*p23*).

week 5

Keep mentally strong. Nothing will sway you off course now – you've come too far for that. Some of the work this week may seem rather testing – the long interval training session in particular. Stay tuned. Put yourself back in the picture. Picture yourself doing the workouts and finishing every one. If you can see it, you can do it!

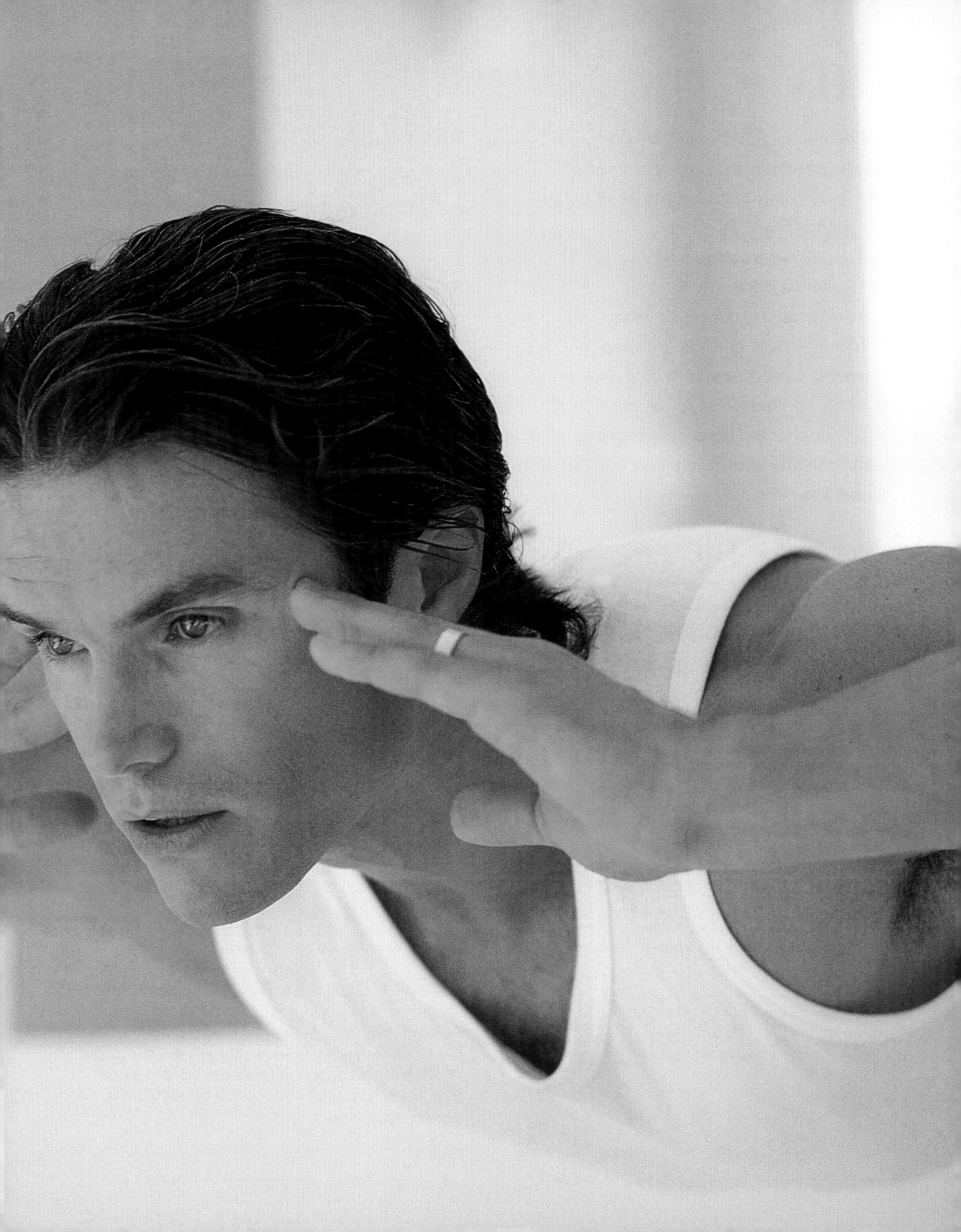

day 29

You've made it past the halfway stage – a time my clients describe as both exciting and nerve-racking. Exciting because you've done so much. The physique you've set your heart on is now in sight. And nerve-racking because you feel there's still a lot to be done.

In a sense, I'd almost be disappointed if you didn't have these feelings. Worrying slightly about achieving your goals is a sign that you're not allowing complacency to set in, that you're still hungry for success. My advice is simple: revisit your goals carefully and make sure you're totally on course with them.

eat & drink

breakfast fresh fruit salad with yogurt and seeds *p132* **or** two slices of whole-wheat toast with nonhydrogenated spread and jam or jelly and a small fruit smoothie *p133*

lunch smoked salmon and dill salad *p138* **or** wild rice salad *p136*

dinner marinated chicken with steamed vegetables *p149* **or** wheat-free pasta with turkey *p148*

snacks apple, pear, 1 oz (25 g) sunflower seeds, 1 oz (25 g) raisins **and** (for men) banana, 1 oz (25 g) sunflower seeds, ½ oz (10 g) raisins

drink at least 2½–3½ pints (1.5–2 liters) of water

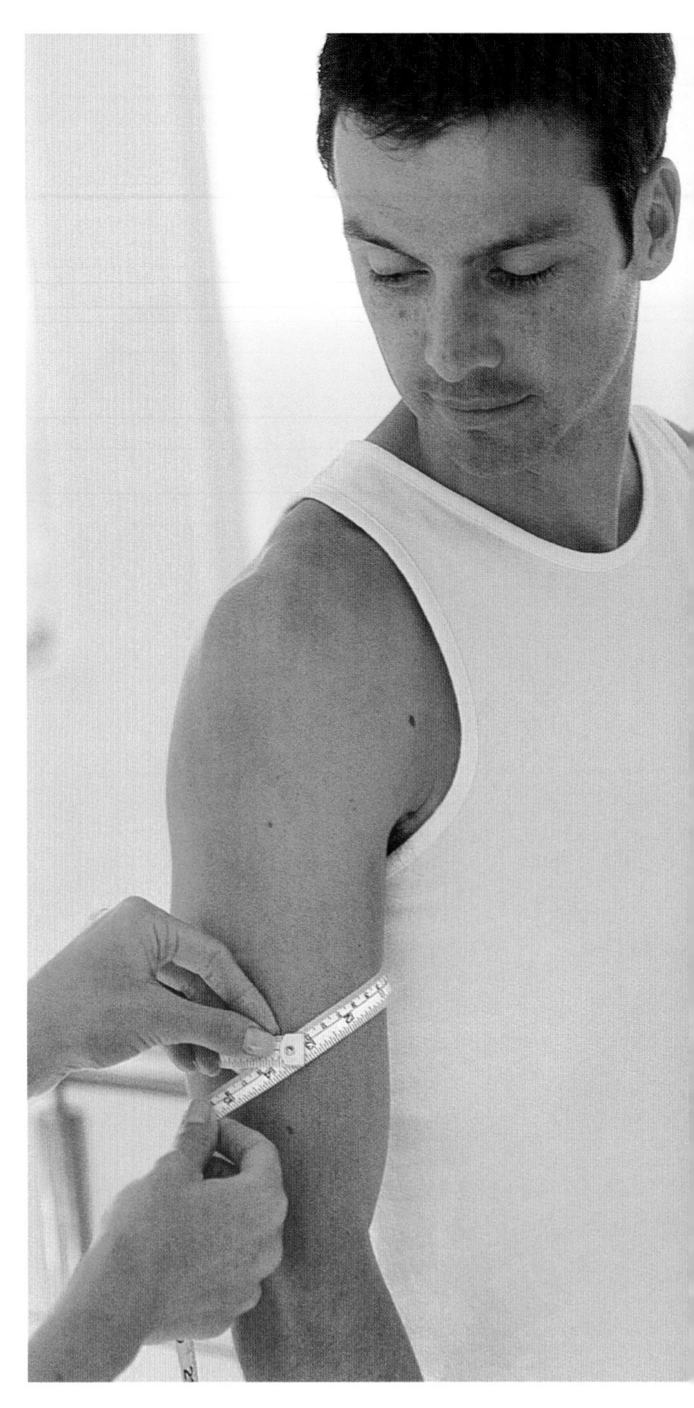

△ You're halfway through, and it's only human nature that you'd like to know how you're getting on. Remember, measuring yourself is a better gauge than weighing yourself – you've lost fat, but you've gained muscle tone.

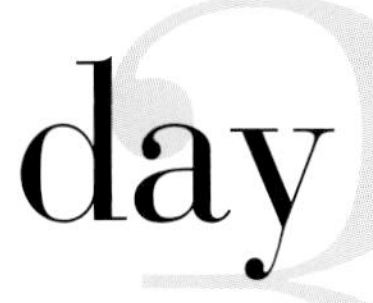

day 30

Just when you thought the workouts were getting easier, all of a sudden they seem difficult again. And they should – I'm taking you up a notch or two.

eat&drink

breakfast wheat-free muesli *p132* **or** oatmeal *p132*

lunch cottage cheese, cranberry and arugula sandwich *p138* **or** broiled vegetable pitas *p139*

dinner baked zucchini with rice *p140* **or** stuffed bell pepper *p142*

snacks apple, pear, and 4 oz (100 g) raspberries or 1 oz (25 g) dried apricots **and** (for men) 1 oz (25 g) mixed sunflower and sesame seeds, 1 oz (25 g) raisins

drink at least 2½–3½ pints (1.5–2 liters) of water

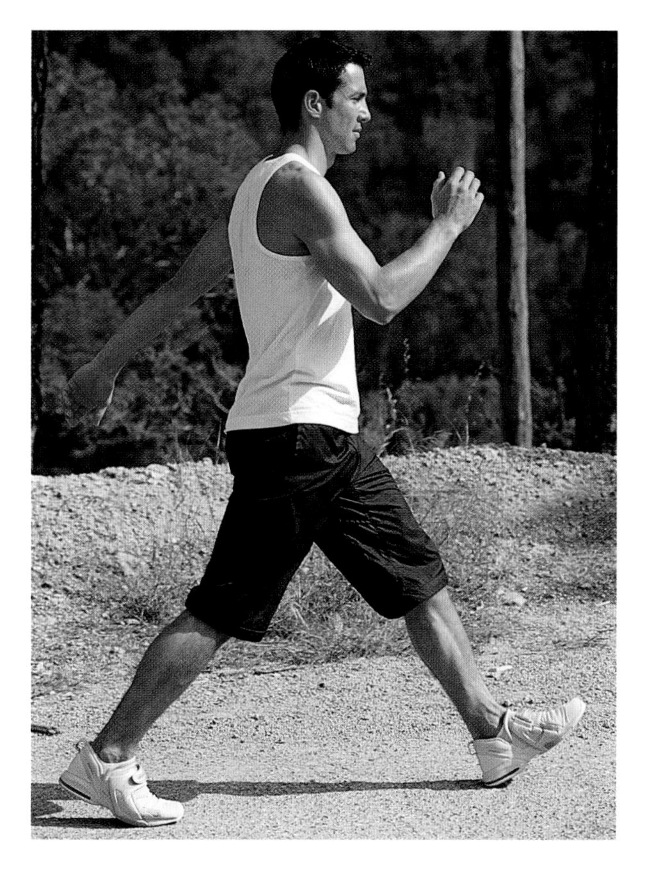

three-part workout

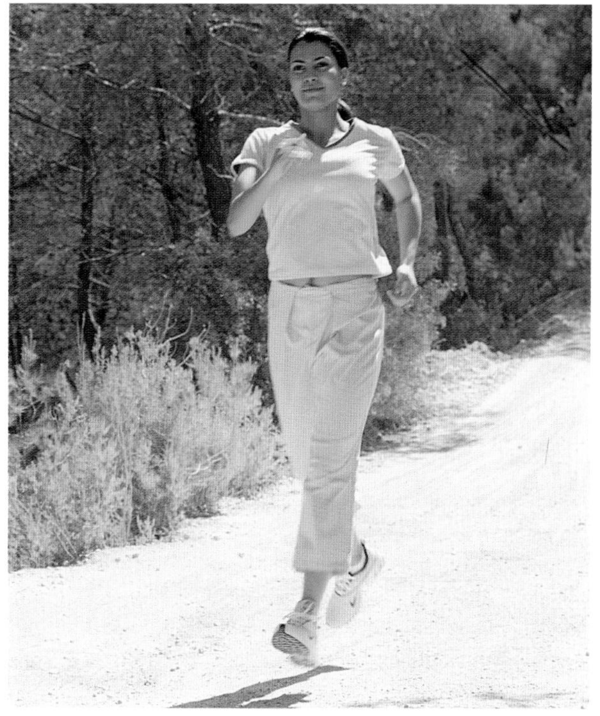

1 cardio

This is the longest interval training session you'll do. The 5-minute intervals will feel particularly intense, so don't go too slowly or they may seem even longer. Fast-pace walk for 3 minutes, then run for 5 minutes. Repeat this three times. Run at 80% MHR (8/10 RPE).

2 resistance

Do the exercises in pairs, so do as many step squats as you can in the specified time, rest for 10 seconds, and then do the same with the body raise. Rest again, then repeat both (with rests). Move on to the next pair. Each pair of exercises (a 'super set') works the front and back of the same limb (or your torso) alternately.

3 stretching

End today's session with a total body stretch (*p22*).

day 30 resistance work

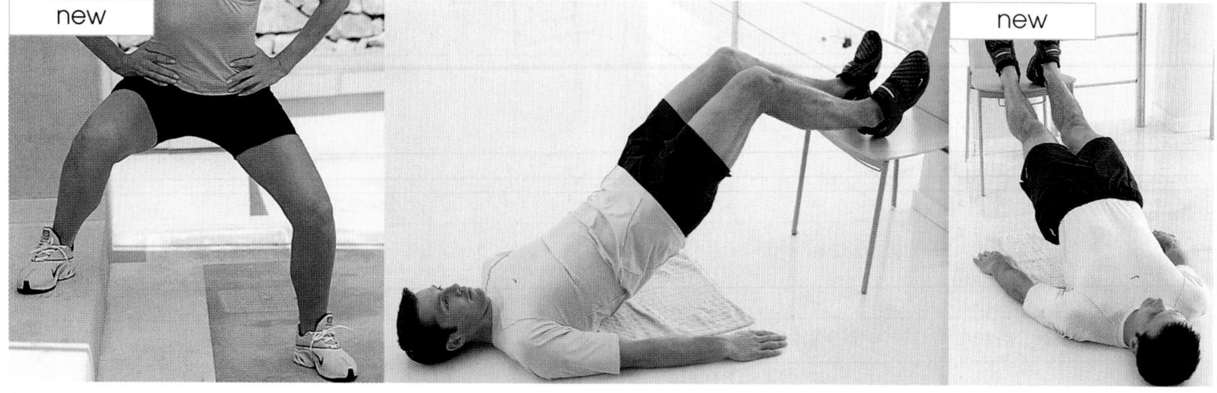

step squat *p87*
① 30 secs per leg ② 45 secs per leg

body raise *p20*
① 30 secs ② 45 secs x2

glute bridge *p87*
① 30 secs ② 45 secs

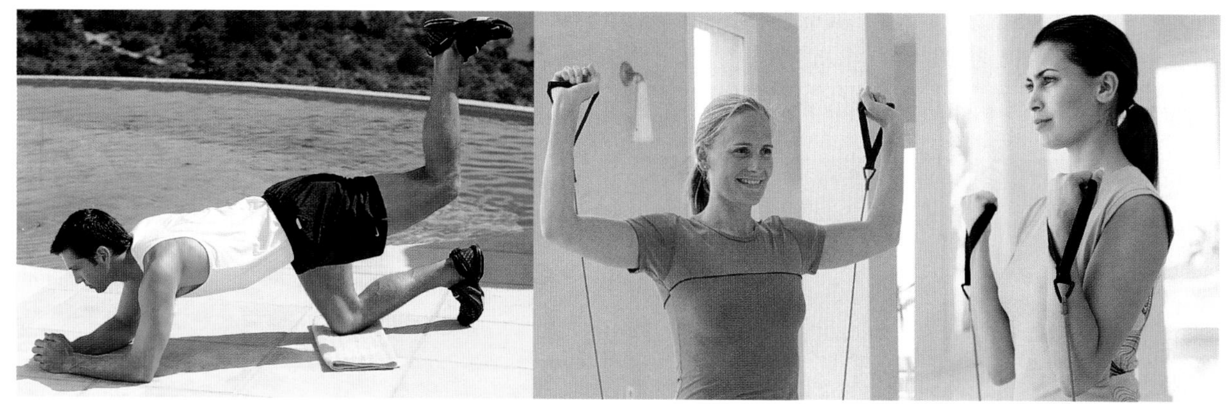

glute raise *p38*
① 30 secs per leg ② 45 secs per leg x2

shoulder press *p52*
① 30 secs ② 45 secs

bicep curl *p21*
① 30 secs ② 45 secs x2

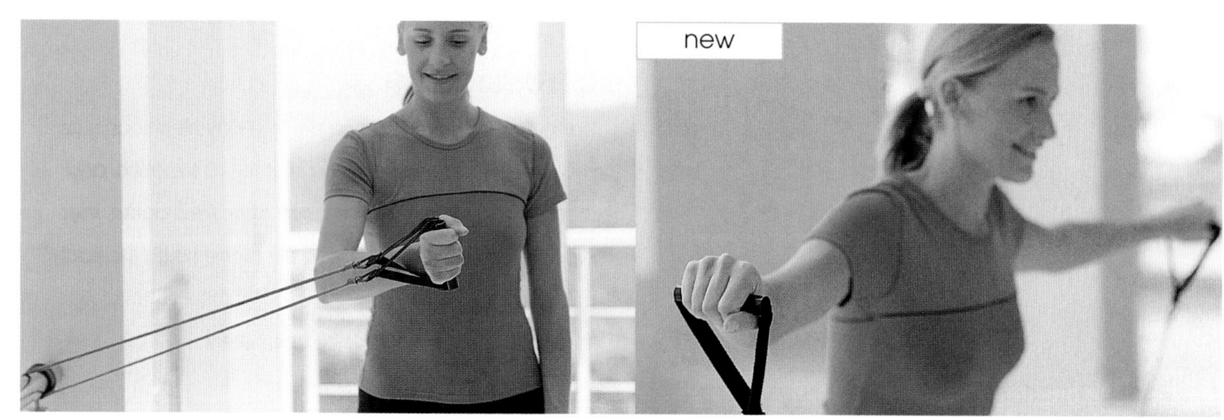

pec fly *p52*
① 30 secs per arm ② 45 secs per arm

bent-over lateral raise *p87*
① 30 secs ② 45 secs x2

day 30 new exercises

bent-over lateral raise ▽

An exercise that's worth doing well, since it tones your upper back and gives definition to the backs of your upper arms.

1 Place your feet hip-width apart on the exertube, knees slightly bent. Wrap the exertube around each foot, then take a handle in each hand. Bend forward slightly, holding the handles at thigh height.

2 Open your arms and lift the handles until they're at shoulder level. Don't tense your neck muscles. Slowly return your arms to the start.

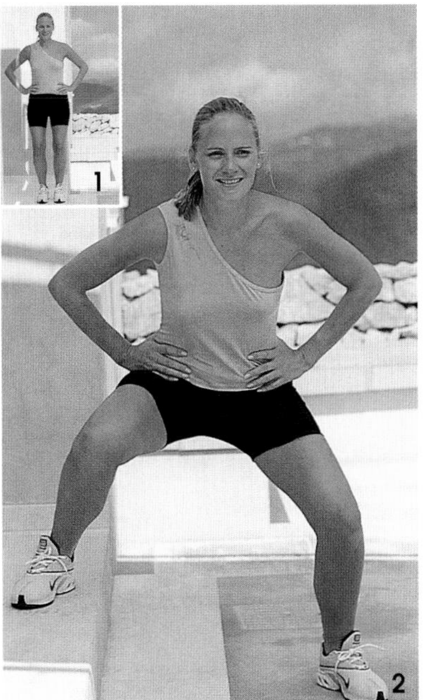

step squat ◁

This is a great way of intensifying the effect of 'basic' squats by putting extra pressure on your working leg.

1 Stand sideways with your feet on a step or stair about 12 in (30 cm) high. Place your hands on your hips.

2 Step sideways off the step. At the same time, bend your knees to 90° and allow your body to lean forward slightly so you adopt a squat position. Make sure you keep your heels on the floor. Return to the start position, using the muscles of the leg on the step.

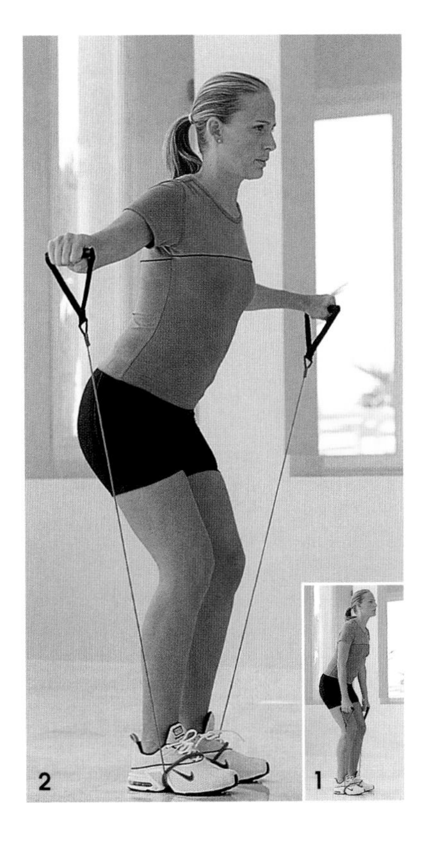

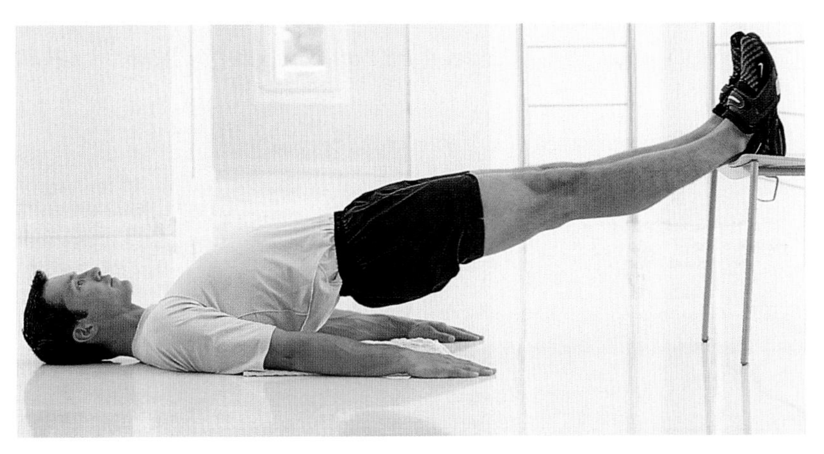

glute bridge △

A fantastic way to tone and shape your bottom, the glute bridge is really a static hold. Focus on controlling it with the muscles of your buttocks.

Lie flat on your back with your heels on a chair. Place your arms by your sides, palms to the floor. Pressing down with your arms, raise your pelvis off the floor until your body is straight from your neck to your toes. Squeeze your buttocks, then slowly lower yourself to the start position.

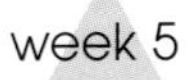

day 31

This has probably been the toughest few days of the plan so far for you. The intensity is high and the heat is on. But it's under this kind of pressure that you can prove yourself – and feel good about doing it. There will be times, however, when for one reason or another you won't be able to work out.

If you do miss a session, you can make up for it. Simply assess what you've missed and add a little extra work to your next workout.

Keep things in proportion, though. If you've missed only one day of the fat loss plan so far, then there's no need to worry about it. If you've missed two or three, you might want to examine your long-term goals.

eat & drink

breakfast whole-wheat pancakes *p132* **or** vegetable omelet *p133*

lunch asparagus and artichoke salad *p135* **or** green salad *p134*

dinner steamed cod with green lentils and tomatoes *p147* **or** monkfish with roasted vegetables *p146*

snacks banana, ½ oz (10 g) almonds, 2 oz (50 g) grapes **and** (for men) apple, and 4 oz (100 g) raspberries or 1 oz (25 g) raisins

drink at least 2½–3½ pints (1.5–2 liters) of water

If you've only **missed one day** of the plan so far, then **don't worry**. If you've missed **two**...

day 32

The resistance part of today's workout is a straight repeat from day 30. I've changed the cardio training slightly, however – I've reduced the length of the intervals, but increased the intensity a little. Make sure that when you're fast-pace walking, you work at a reasonably high heart rate.

eat & drink

breakfast fresh fruit salad with yogurt and seeds *p132* **or** large fruit smoothie *p133*

lunch quinoa salad *p136* **or** Camargue rice salad *p136*

dinner carrot and sweet potato fishcakes with herb salad *p144* **or** steamed fish with salsa and salad *p144*

snacks apple, pear, 1 oz (25 g) sunflower seeds, 1 oz (25 g) raisins **and** (for men) banana, 1 oz (25 g) sunflower seeds, ½ oz (10 g) raisins

drink at least 2½–3½ pints (1.5–2 liters) of water

three-part workout

Fast-pace walk for 90 seconds, then run for 3 minutes. Repeat five times so that you walk and run a total of six times. Run at 85% MHR (8–9/10 RPE). Move on to the resistance work and repeat the super set training from day 30. Finish the session with a total body stretch (*p22*).

day 33

Regular stretching should take care of most of your muscle aches and pains. But on a rest day you could probably handle a little pampering. A massage may be just what you need.

Massage relaxes your muscles and improves your circulation. The psychological benefits are important, too – you'll feel pampered, cared for, and know your body is worth all the effort.

Unless you're having a specific problem, you don't need to see a qualified therapist (though this could make the experience far more enjoyable). You can either massage yourself or call upon the help of a friend or partner. A few drops of aromatic oil will greatly enhance the effect.

eat&drink

breakfast wheat-free muesli *p132* **or** oatmeal *p132*

lunch salade niçoise *p137* **or** Greek salad *p134*

dinner marinated tuna with polenta *p145*
or wheat-free pasta with tomato and shrimp sauce *p148*

snacks apple, pear, and 4 oz (100 g) raspberries or 1 oz (25 g) dried apricots **and** (for men) 1 oz (25 g) mixed sunflower and sesame seeds, 1 oz (25 g) raisins

drink at least 2½–3½ pints (1.5–2 liters) of water

▽ A combination of stroking, rubbing, and kneading will relieve tension from both body and mind, and make tight, sore muscles supple again. See it as your rest day treat.

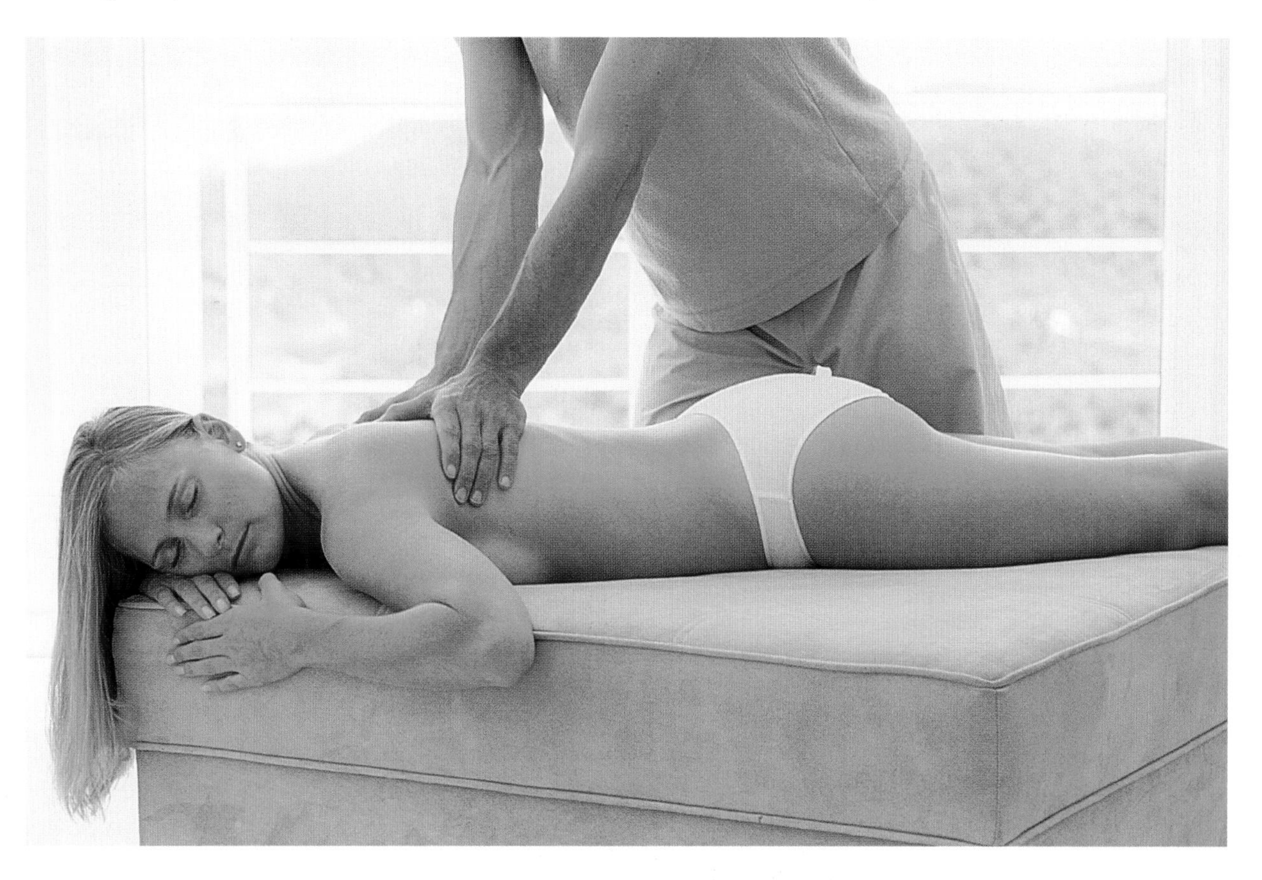

day 34

Both the cardio and resistance parts of today's workout should get you good and hot and sweaty, since my aim is to raise your metabolic rate significantly. They'll also leave you very hungry, so make sure you plan your meal times carefully.

During the cardio session, short fast intervals, with little recovery time, will have you breathing hard and feeling as if you're using your muscles hard, too. Make sure your breathing is strong and that you're working at the right level.

More super sets for you to do in the resistance session mean this a tough workout. As your body starts to tire, keep an eye on your technique.

eat&drink

breakfast poached egg on two slices of dry whole-wheat toast **or** whole-wheat pancakes *p132*

lunch smoked salmon and dill salad *p138* **or** wild rice salad *p136*

dinner lemon shrimp with three bean salad *p148* **or** Asian stir fry *p141*

snacks banana, ½ oz (10 g) almonds, 2 oz (50 g) grapes **and** (for men) apple, and 4 oz (100 g) raspberries or 1 oz (25 g) raisins

drink at least 2½–3½ pints (1.5–2 liters) of water

three-part workout

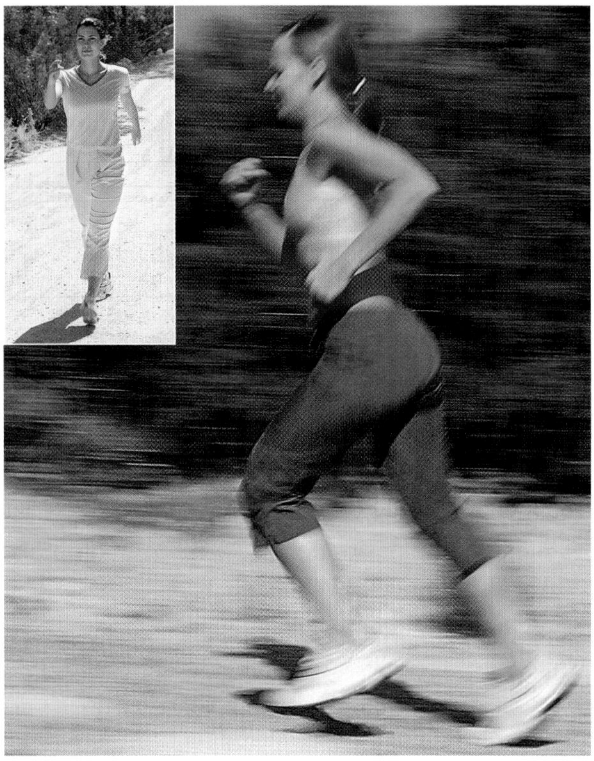

1 cardio

For the interval work today, fast-pace walk for 1 minute, then run for 1 minute. Repeat this seven times. Run at 90% MHR (9/10 RPE).

2 resistance

The resistance work today is super sets. Unlike day 30, this time I'd like you to perform the number of reps indicated. The first four exercises are your first super set, so perform them in order, with 10-second rests in between. Then repeat them in order twice (with rests), with a 30-second rest between sets. The last four exercises are your second super set. Do them in the same way.

3 stretching

Finish your workout with a short standing stretch (*p23*).

day 34 resistance work

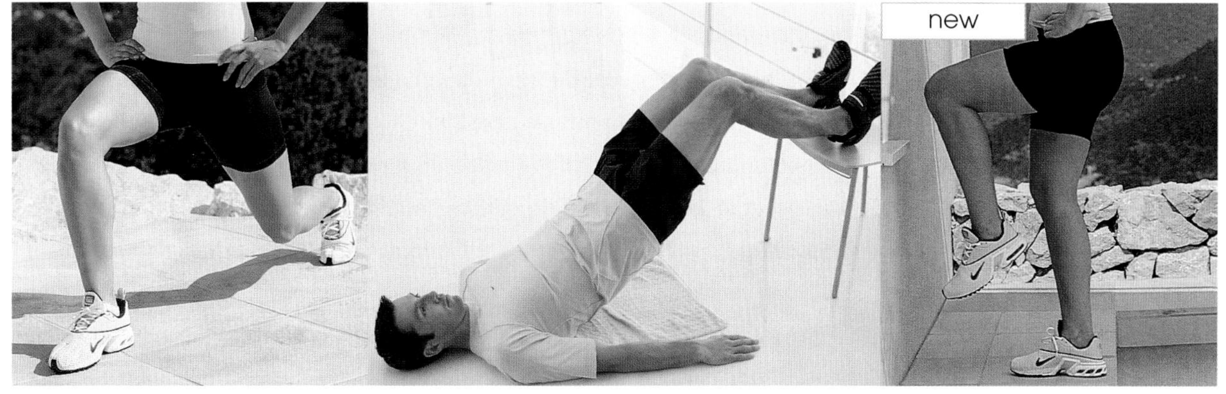

power lunge *p75*
① 12 reps per leg ② 15 reps per leg

body raise *p20*
① 20 reps ② 25 reps

knee raise *p92*
① 15 reps per leg ② 20 reps per leg

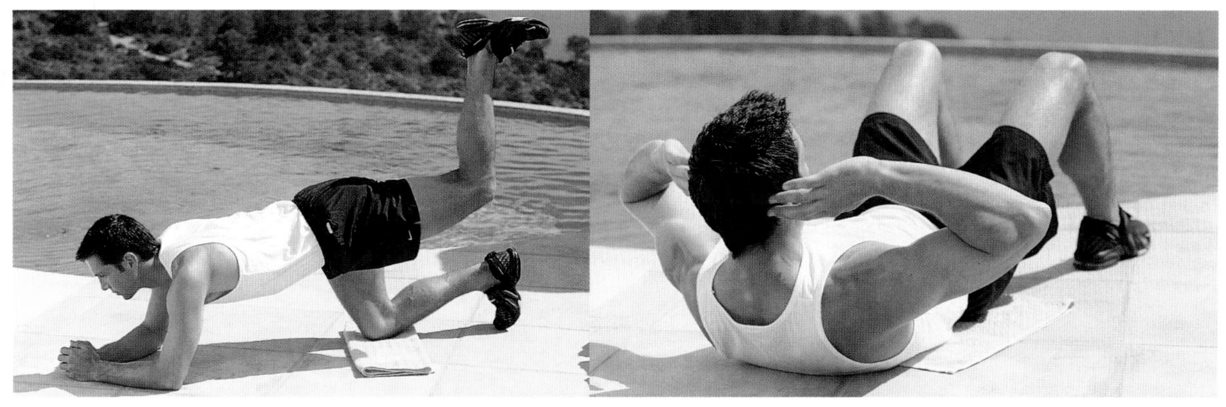

glute raise *p38*
① 20 reps per leg ② 25 reps per leg x3

crunch *p21*
① 20 reps ② 30 reps

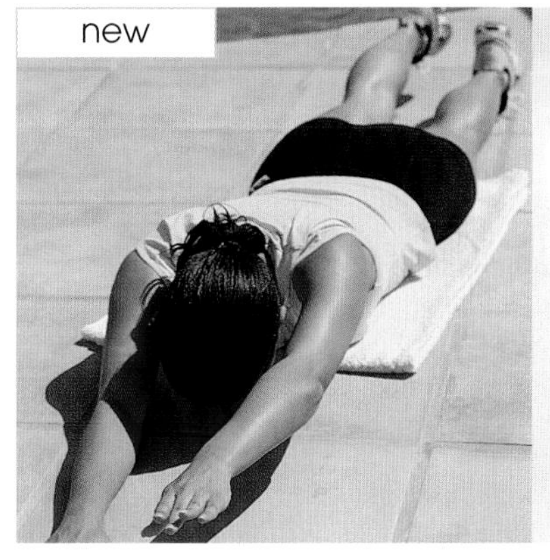

dorsal raise *p92*
① & ② 20 reps per side

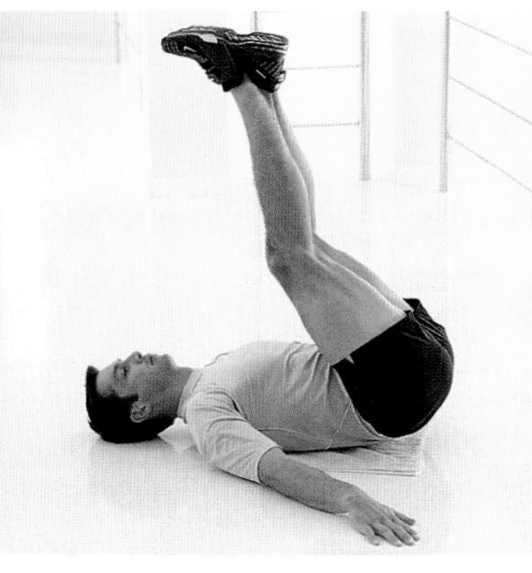

reverse curl *p43*
① 15 reps ② 20 reps

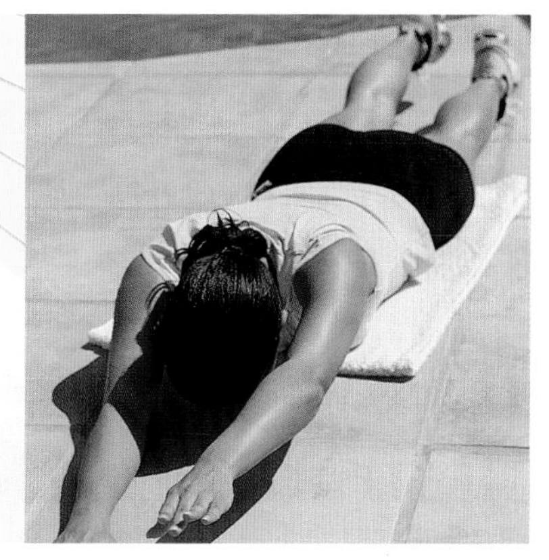

dorsal raise *p92*
① & ② 20 reps per side x3

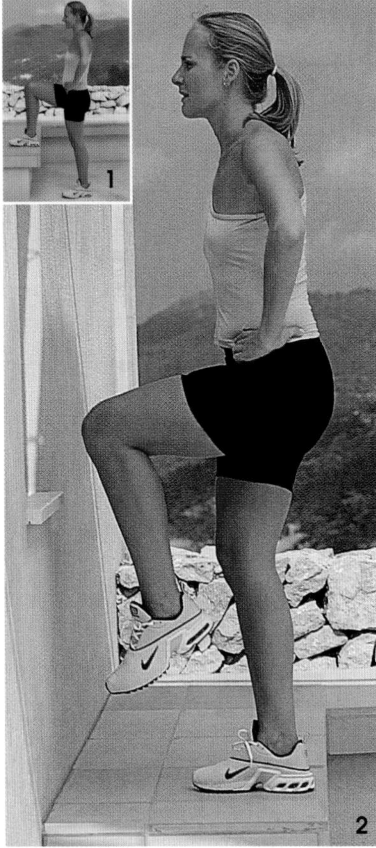

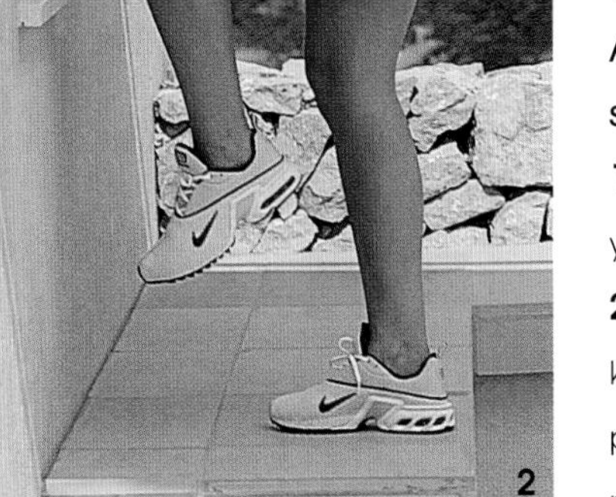

knee raise ◁

A lower body exercise that works as many of the muscles of your legs in as many directions as possible.

1 Stand facing a step or stair about 16 in (40 cm) high. Place one foot on the step, but keep the other one on the floor. Place your hands on your hips.

2 Step up with your other foot, but instead of placing your foot on the step, raise your knee straight to hip height. Lower your knee and place your foot on the floor again. Step down to the start position, your leading foot first.

dorsal raise ▽

An exercise derived from Pilates, the dorsal raise improves posture by strengthening the muscles that run along the lower part of your spine.

1 Lie on your front on a mat with your arms stretched out in front of you and your legs straight. Be careful not to tense the muscles of your neck.

2 Breathe out. At the same time, raise one arm and your opposite leg. Try to keep them both straight. Hold for 1 second, then slowly lower them to the start position, breathing in as you do so. Work your opposite arm and leg when you perform the next rep.

The knee raise is a dynamic exercise that will test your thighs and bottom hard.

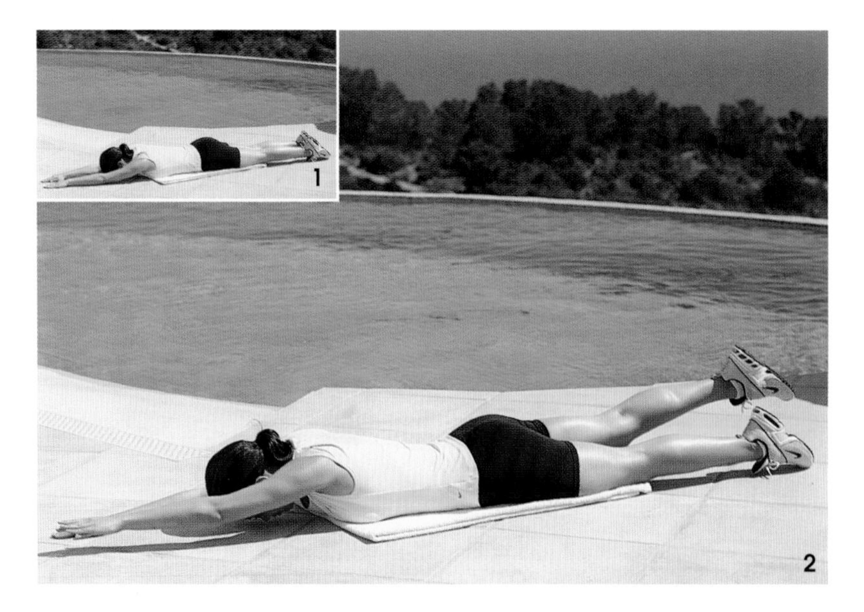

day 35

This is another 'cardio only' day, and although the session is 45 minutes long, you should actually find it pretty straightforward.

Exercising with a friend or partner can transform these long cardio sessions. Not only will you have someone to keep you company and encourage you if necessary, but it's also interesting to have a person with a different exercise style or speed right next to you.

eat&drink

breakfast fresh fruit salad with yogurt and seeds *p132* **or** oatmeal *p132*

lunch cottage cheese, cranberry and arugula sandwich *p138* **or** broiled vegetable pitas *p139*

dinner smoked salmon and lentil salad *p147* **or** vegetable and tofu kabobs *p142*

snacks apple, pear, 1 oz (25 g) sunflower seeds, 1 oz (25 g) raisins **and** (for men) banana, 1 oz (25 g) sunflower seeds, ½ oz (10 g) raisins

drink at least 2½–3½ pints (1.5–2 liters) of water

If you tend to take the **same route** for your run or fast-pace walk, try to **find another** so you push your body through **fresh challenges.**

two-part workout

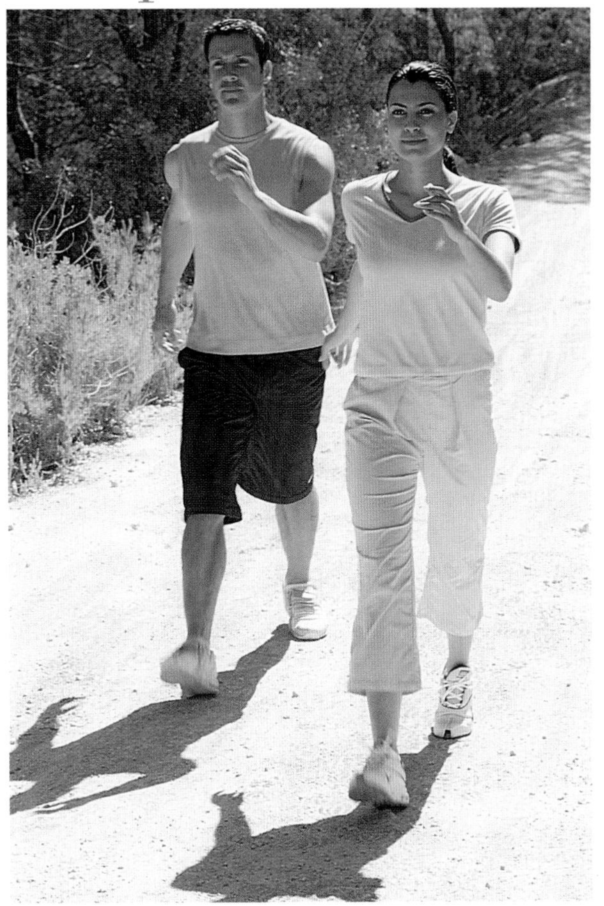

1 cardio

Run or fast-pace walk at a constant pace for 45 minutes. Work at 70–75% MHR (7–8/10 RPE).

2 stretching

Round off today's 'cardio only' workout with a lower body stretch (*p23*). If the weather's nice, you could do it outside, right after your run or walk.

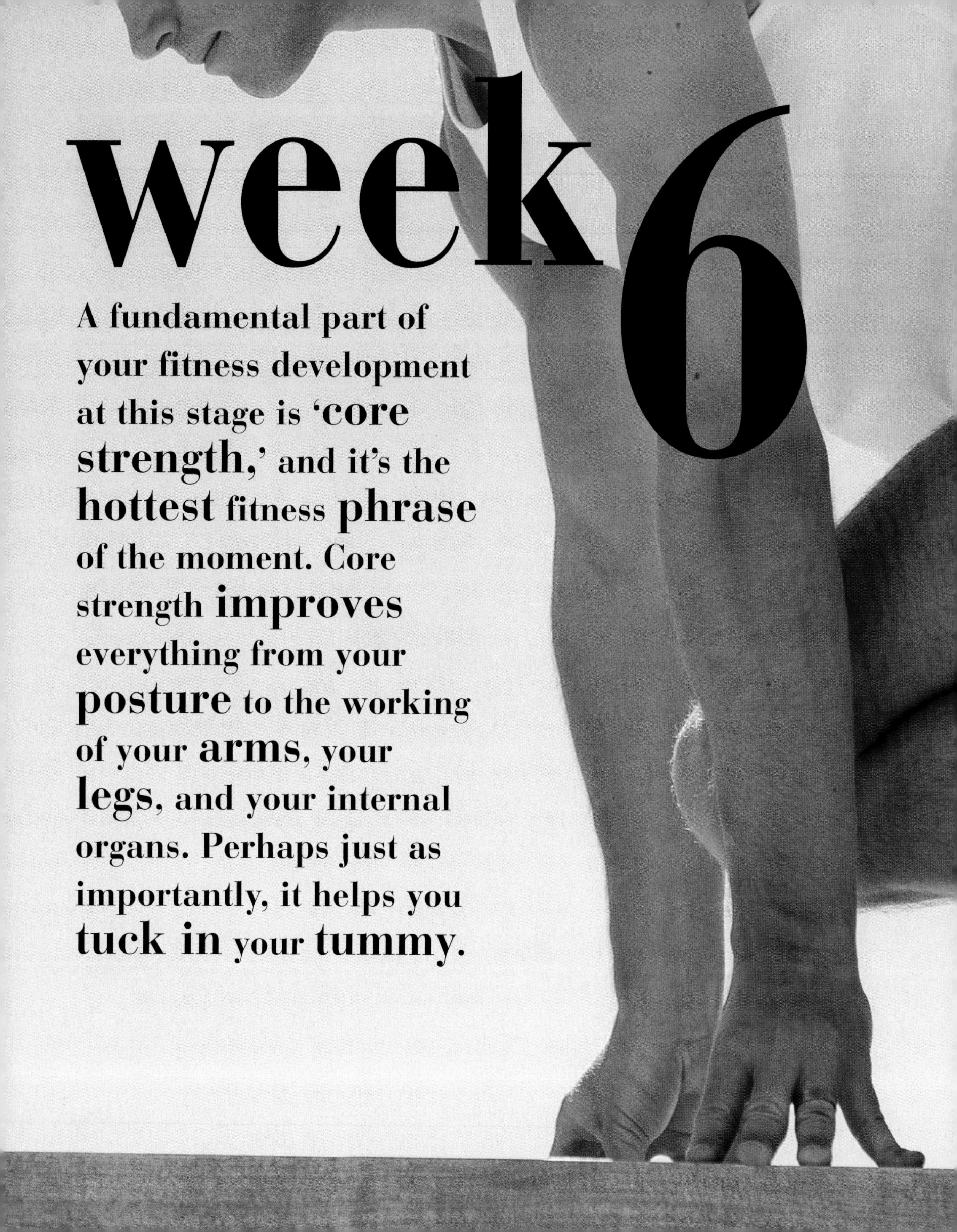

week 6

A fundamental part of your fitness development at this stage is 'core strength,' and it's the hottest fitness phrase of the moment. Core strength improves everything from your posture to the working of your arms, your legs, and your internal organs. Perhaps just as importantly, it helps you tuck in your tummy.

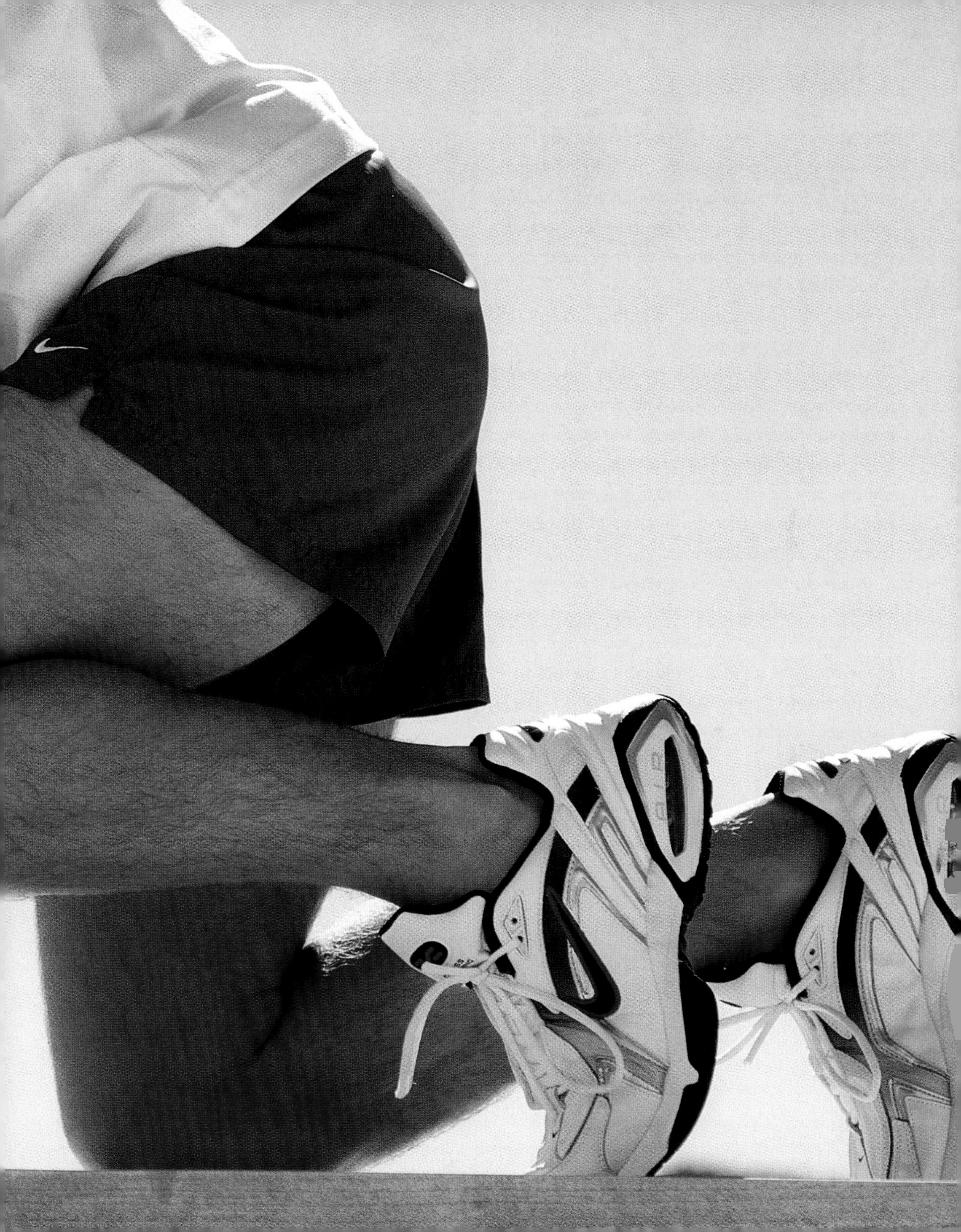

day 36

One phrase that's been overused recently by fitness professionals is 'core strength.' It's actually nothing new, but has certainly been brought to the public's attention in a big way over the past few years. So, what do people mean when they talk about creating core strength?

Well, they're actually referring to all the important muscles around your spine and the related areas of your body. With good core strength, your posture is improved and your internal organs function more efficiently. You have a good base level of fitness that you can put to use in almost any sport. Better still, you have strong stomach muscles that are needed to support the spine and avoid back pain.

There are any number of ways of creating core strength – many of which can seem rather complicated – but the exercises you're performing at the moment are doing the job to perfection. At the same time, they're pushing you toward your fat loss goal. Flat tummy, here you come.

eat & drink

breakfast wheat-free muesli *p132* **or** two slices of whole-wheat toast with nonhydrogenated spread and jam or jelly

lunch asparagus and artichoke salad *p135* **or** green salad *p134*

dinner sweet potato gnocchi with tomato and shrimp sauce *p140* **or** steamed fish with Moroccan vegetables *p146*

snacks apple, pear, and 4 oz (100 g) raspberries or 1 oz (25 g) dried apricots **and** (for men) 1 oz (25 g) mixed sunflower and sesame seeds, 1 oz (25 g) raisins

drink at least 2½–3½ pints (1.5–2 liters) of water

day 37

Once again, the cardio training should be pretty straightforward for you today. The resistance work, on the other hand, might seem rather tough.

Your cardio fitness has improved greatly over the past few weeks – and so has your ability to cope with the resistance work. Which is why I want to push you with a tougher session now.

eat & drink

breakfast poached egg on two slices of dry whole-wheat toast **or** whole-wheat pancakes *p132*

lunch salade niçoise *p137* **or** Greek salad *p134*

dinner broiled fish with sweet potato and spinach bake *p144* **or** marinated chicken with steamed vegetables *p149*

snacks banana, ½ oz (10 g) almonds, 2 oz (50 g) grapes **and** (for men) apple, and 4 oz (100 g) raspberries or 1 oz (25 g) raisins

drink at least 2½–3½ pints (1.5–2 liters) of water

three-part workout

1 cardio

Run or fast-pace walk at a constant pace for 30 minutes. Work at 75–80% MHR (7–8/10 RPE).

2 resistance

The resistance work for today is based on compound training (*p60*). Perform the reps for the first four exercises, rest for 1 minute, then repeat. Rest, then perform the next three exercises in exactly the same way. Finally, repeat the process with the last four exercises.

3 stretching

Finish the workout with a total body stretch (*p22*).

day 37 resistance work

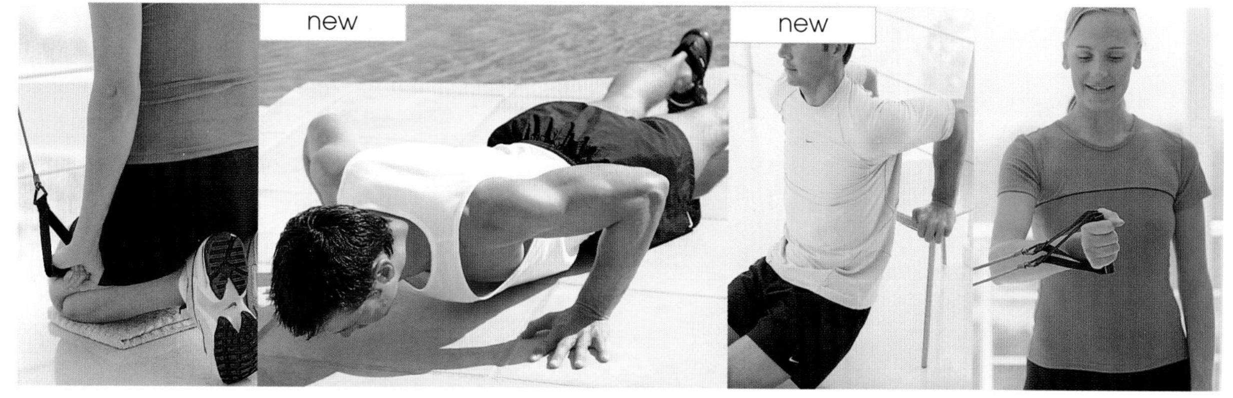

tricep press *p56*
① & ② 15 reps

push-up *p98*
① 10 reps ② 12 reps

advanced dip *p98*
① 15 reps ② 20 reps

pec fly *p52*
① & ② 12 reps per arm x2

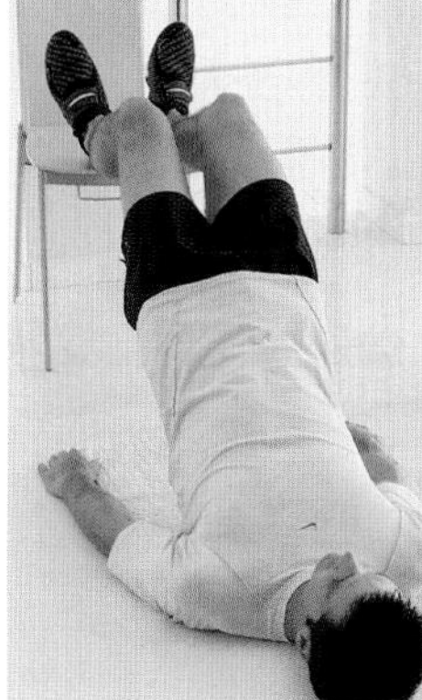

body raise *p20*
① & ② 20 reps

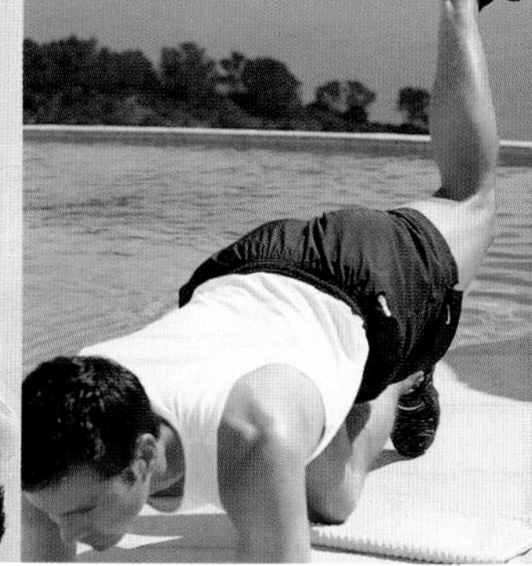

glute raise *p38*
① 20 per leg ② 20 per leg

walking lunge *p75*
① & ② 20 strides x2

crunch *p21*
① 30 reps ② 40 reps

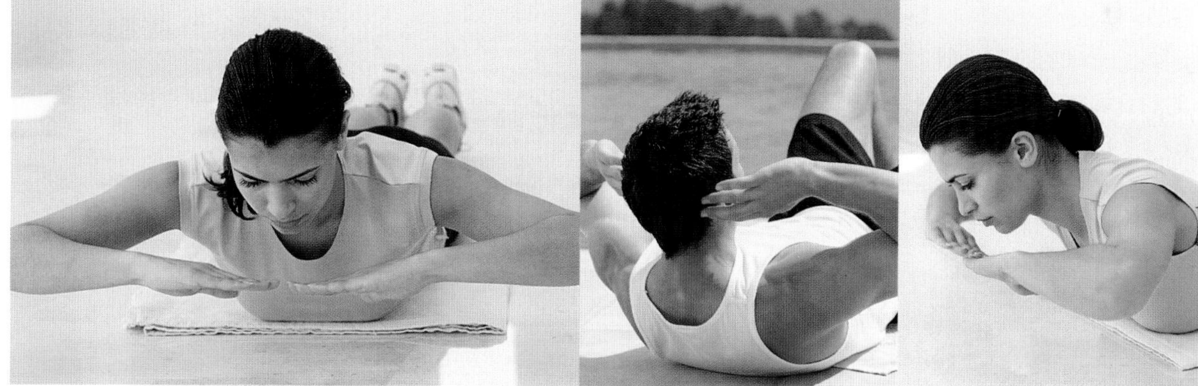

back extension *p38*
① 20 reps ② 20 reps

crunch *p21*
① 30 reps ② 40 reps

back extension *p38*
① 20 reps ② 20 reps x2

day 37 new exercises

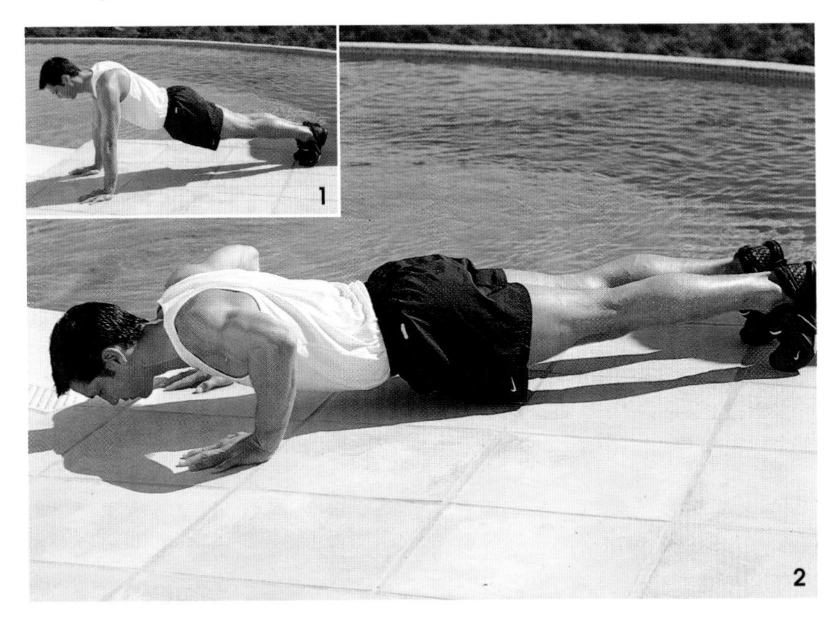

push-up ◁

Push-ups use the weight of the body to work your chest, arm, and shoulder muscles.

1 Place your hands under your shoulders, fingers pointing forward. Keep your legs and body straight, and your feet hip-width apart.

2 Breathe in and bend your arms to about 90°, lowering your body as you do so. Keep your head in line with your spine, and your tummy and thigh muscles tight. Breathe out as you push back up to the start.

advanced dip ▷

More difficult than the 'basic' dip, the advanced dip gives you rapid development by working your arm, chest, and shoulder muscles more effectively.

1 Place the palms of your hands on the corners of a chair, so you're supporting your upper body weight with your arms. Keep your back straight and close to the chair. Slowly extend your legs in front of you, keeping them hip-width apart.

2 Keeping your body close to the chair at all times, lower yourself down until your arms are bent behind you at 90°. Push up with your arms to return to the start position – your arms should be straight but not locked.

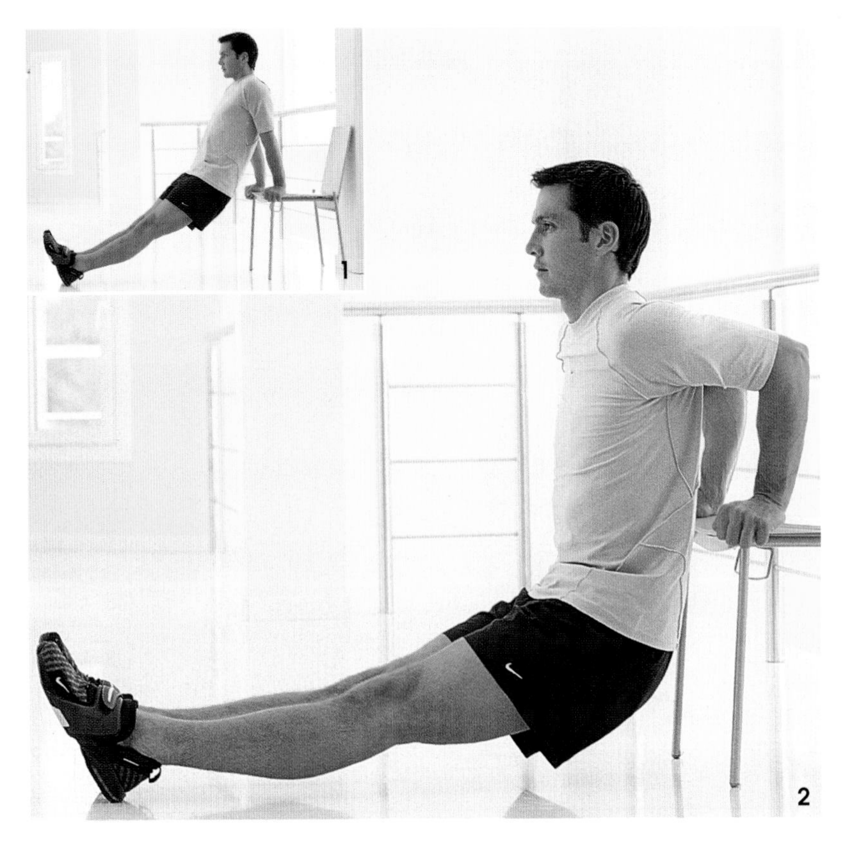

day 38

When I was putting together the fat loss plan diet for you, I decided to reduce the intake of two of the most common causes of food intolerances – that's wheat and dairy products.

An estimated 90% of people suffer from food intolerances, which affect their lives in some way or other. Symptoms can range from lethargy, headaches, asthma, and eczema to arthritis, difficulty losing weight, and obesity.

Food intolerances occur when the body finds it difficult to digest a food and produces toxic by-products as it attempts to break it down. Some food intolerances are permanent – if your body has always found a particular food difficult to digest, it probably always will. Dairy products, shrimp, and peanuts are common culprits. Identifying the food and either reducing your intake of it or eliminating it altogether can have a profound and positive effect on your general health.

It's also possible to develop a food intolerance. This often happens with foods like wheat that we tend to rely too heavily upon. In this case, there's no need to eliminate the food permanently, but a temporary break from it is beneficial. I've opted for a halfway measure.

eat&drink

breakfast wheat-free muesli *p132* **or** oatmeal *p132*

lunch smoked salmon and dill salad *p138*
or asparagus and artichoke salad *p135*

dinner broiled or steamed fish with quinoa *p143*
or chicken with couscous and mint yogurt *p149*

snacks apple, pear, 1 oz (25 g) sunflower seeds, 1 oz (25 g) raisins **and** (for men) banana, 1 oz (25 g) sunflower seeds, ½ oz (10 g) raisins

drink at least 2½–3½ pints (1.5–2 liters) of water

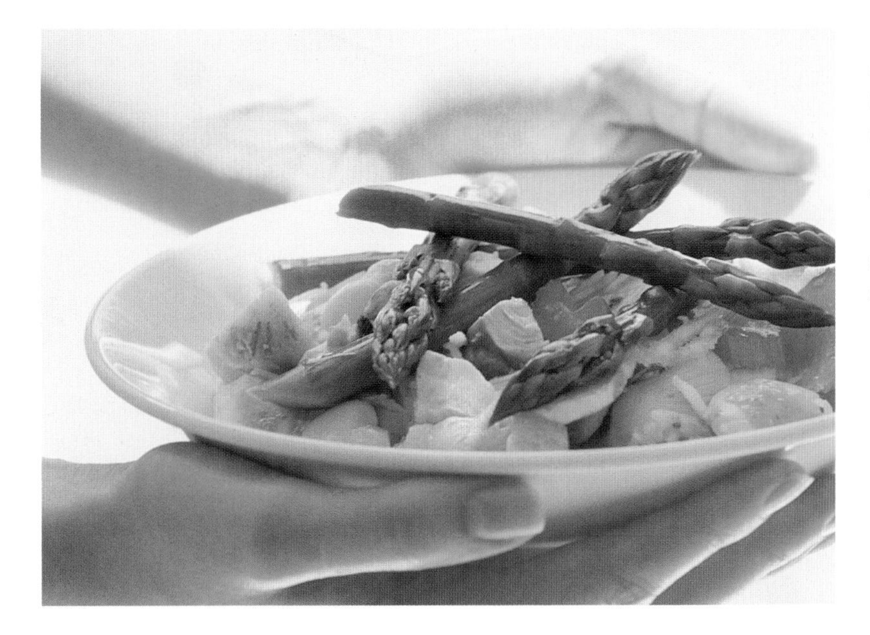

◁ An intolerance to wheat is common, so on the fat loss plan you have a reduced intake – only one meal per day at most contains it. In place of a sandwich at lunchtime, for instance, you can enjoy meals like this asparagus and artichoke salad (*p135*), which is healthy, sustaining, and delicious.

day 39

After a day's rest, you should feel all set to attack today's session with gusto. It's a repeat of day 37, but I'd like you to give an extra 5% on the cardio work. Remind yourself of the gains you'll make from demanding more.

eat & drink

breakfast fresh fruit salad with yogurt and seeds *p132* **or** raspberry fool *p132*

lunch broiled vegetable pitas *p139* **or** cottage cheese, cranberry and arugula sandwich *p138*

dinner monkfish with roasted vegetables *p146* **or** mushroom risotto *p142*

snacks apple, pear, and 4 oz (100 g) raspberries or 1 oz (25 g) dried apricots **and** (for men) 1 oz (25 g) mixed sunflower and sesame seeds, 1 oz (25 g) raisins

drink at least 2½–3½ pints (1.5–2 liters) of water

three-part workout

Perform the same workout as on day 37. But for the cardio, increase the rate you work at to 80–85% MHR (8–9/10 RPE). As before, finish the workout by doing a total body stretch (*p22*).

day 40

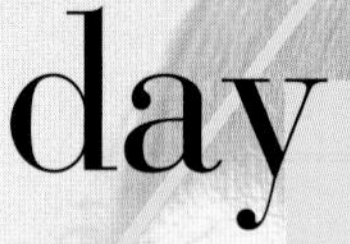

Earlier in the plan (on day 8), I gave you some ways of speeding up your metabolic rate by increasing your daily acitivity level. It's this, you'll remember, that often makes a difference between losing weight and retaining it.

You've doubtless had ideas of your own since then, but let me give you some more of mine.

- Whenever possible, leave your car at home and walk instead.
- If you travel by public transportation, get off at a station or stop before you need to and walk the rest.
- Cancel your newspaper delivery and walk to the store or vending box every day to buy a copy.
- If you have a message to deliver in the office, 'walk' it over rather than emailing it.
- Dive into that spring-cleaning you've been promising yourself you'll do. And do it energetically. Or take yourself out to your garden – just 10 minutes of digging burns 80 calories. Even weeding, you'll expend about 35 calories.

Cultivate good habits: it's that simple.

eat & drink

breakfast wheat-free muesli *p132* **or** two slices of whole-wheat toast with nonhydrogenated spread and jam or jelly

lunch asparagus and artichoke salad *p135* **or** Camargue rice salad *p136*

dinner Thai-style vegetables with polenta *p141* **or** carrot and sweet potato fishcakes with herb salad *p144*

snacks banana, ½ oz (10 g) almonds, 2 oz (50 g) grapes **and** (for men) apple, and 4 oz (100 g) raspberries or 1 oz (25 g) raisins

drink at least 2½–3½ pints (1.5–2 liters) of water

day 41

Today is the first of two back-to-back exercise days that will be the toughest of the whole plan. They take a little longer than the others, too, so plan your days in a way that gives you some extra time.

The cardio is a long but moderate session that will burn a lot of fat. Whether you're running, fast-pace walking, or cycling, try to find yourself a different route – it will push your body through fresh challenges.

eat&drink

breakfast poached egg on two slices of dry whole-wheat toast **or** whole-wheat pancakes *p132*

lunch quinoa salad *p136* **or** wild rice salad *p136*

dinner baked zucchini with rice *p140* **or** marinated tuna with polenta *p145*

snacks apple, pear, 1 oz (25 g) sunflower seeds, 1 oz (25 g) raisins **and** (for men) banana, 1 oz (25 g) sunflower seeds, ½ oz (10 g) raisins

drink at least 2½–3½ pints (1.5–2 liters) of water

This is the first of two back-to-back exercise days that are going to be the toughest part of the whole plan.

three-part workout

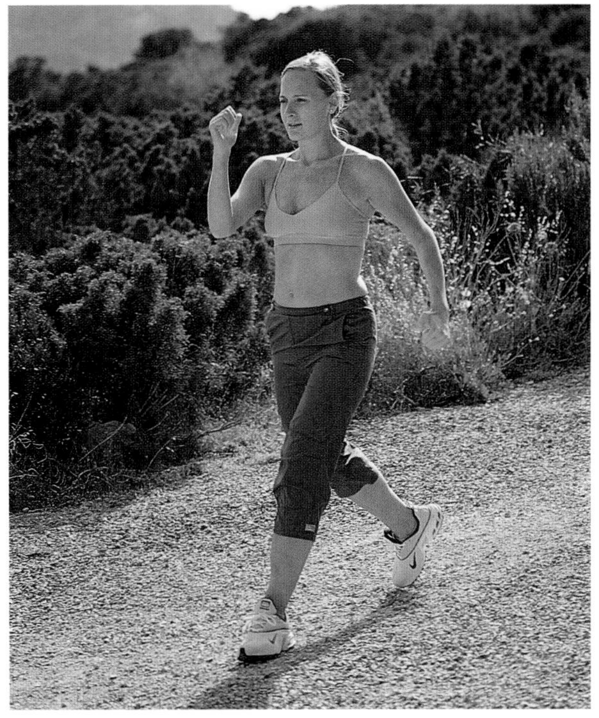

1 cardio

Run or fast-pace walk at a constant pace for 45 minutes. Work at 80% MHR (8/10 RPE).

2 resistance

The resistance work for today is more PHA (peripheral heart action), which works your upper and lower body alternately. Peform the reps for the exercises in order, resting for 10 seconds between each exercise. After the last exercise (the pec fly), rest for 2 minutes, and then repeat the whole process. Level ② users, make sure there is plenty of resistance on your exertube (*see day 9*).

3 stretching

End this long workout by performing a short standing stretch (*p23*). If you have the time, take it slowly so you relax your muscles well.

day 41 resistance work

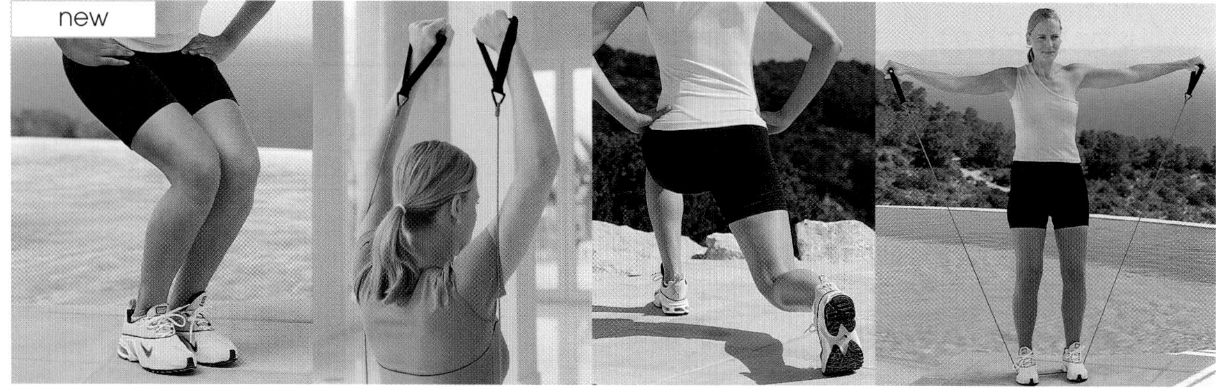

close squat *p103*
① 20 reps ② 25 reps

shoulder press *p52*
① 15 reps ② 25 reps

walking lunge *p75*
① & ② 20 strides

lateral raise *p21*
① 15 reps ② 15 reps

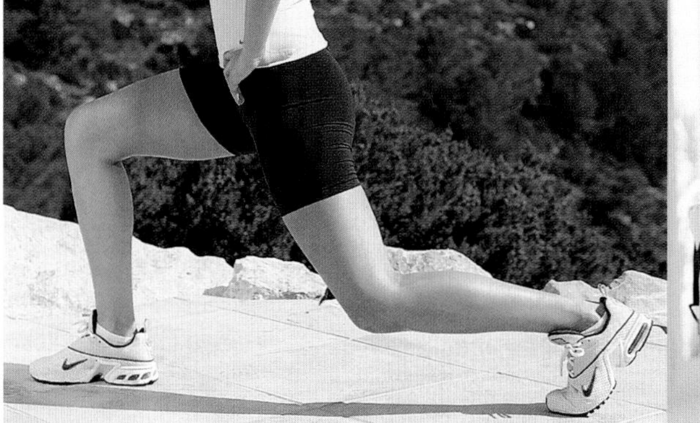

power lunge *p75*
① 15 reps per leg ② 15 reps per leg

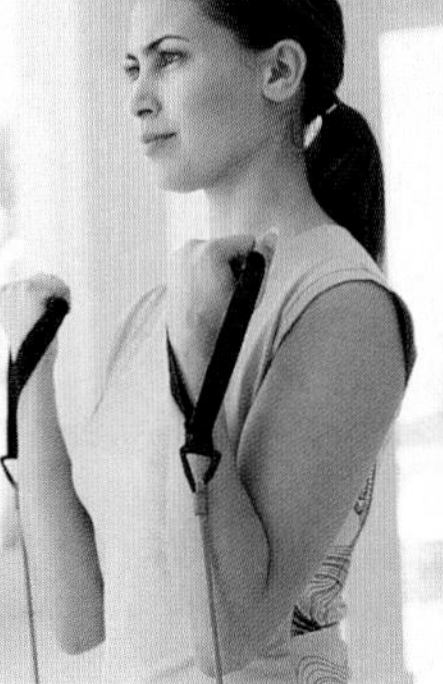

bicep curl *p21*
① 20 reps ② 12 reps

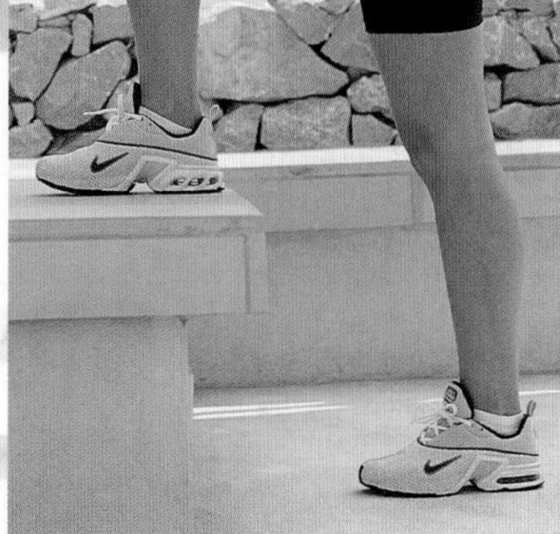

step-up *p62*
① 15 reps per leg ② 20 reps per leg

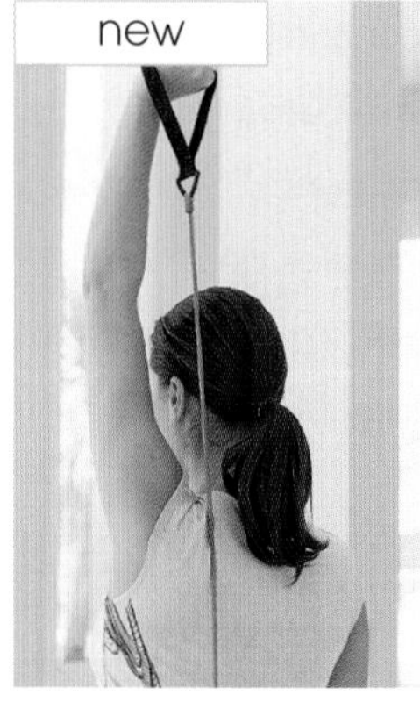

tricep overhead *p103*
① & ② 15 reps per arm

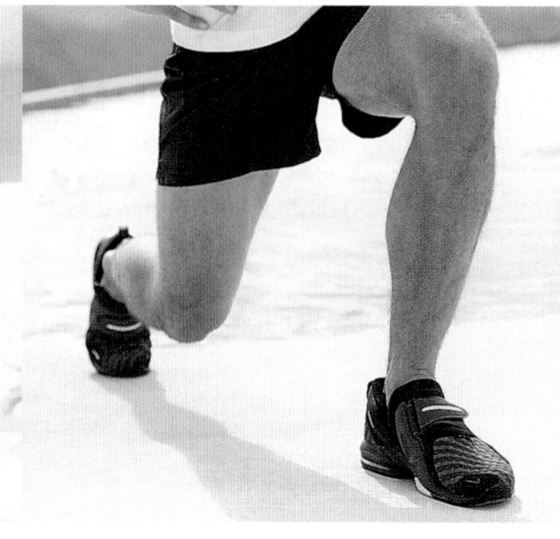

lunge *p56*
① 15 reps per leg ② 25 reps per leg

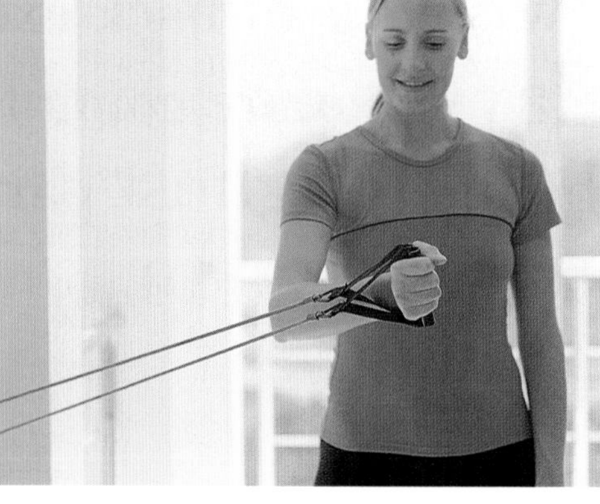

pec fly *p52*
① 12 reps per arm ② 15 reps per arm x2

day 41 new exercises

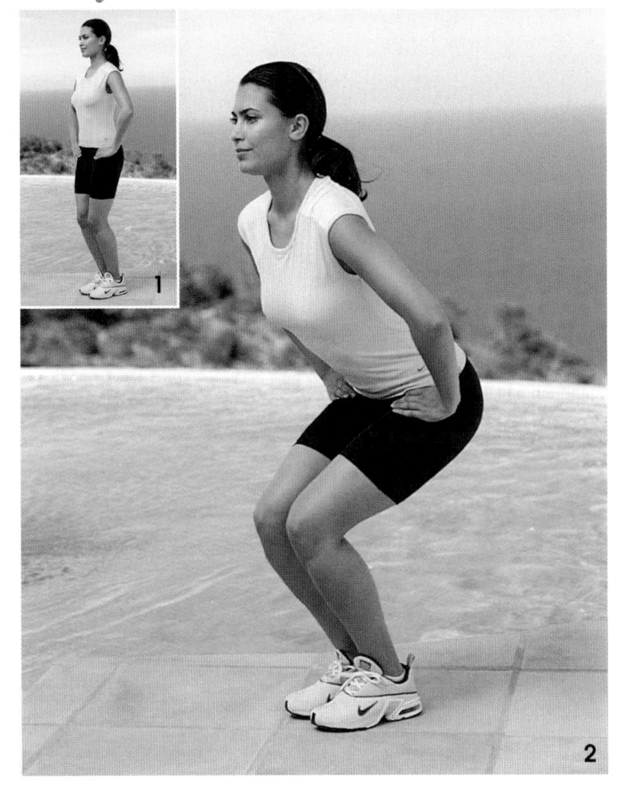

close squat ◁

This puts intensive pressure on your buttocks, as well as working your thighs the way all squats do.

1 Stand with your feet together and your knees slightly bent. Keep your back straight and your tummy pulled in. Place your hands on the top of your thighs.

2 Imagine you're sitting back on a chair, then bend your knees to 90° and lower your body until it's at right angles to your thighs. Keep your body weight through the heels of your feet, and make sure your knees don't go beyond your toes. Slowly raise yourself to the start position.

tricep overhead ▷

A simple but effective way to work the muscles on the backs of your upper arms.

1 Place one foot about two-thirds of the way along the exertube, with the handle of the long end in one hand. Plant your other foot a step's-length forward and bend your knee slightly. Rest your other hand on the top of your thigh, and put your body weight on the heel of your front foot. Keeping your back straight and your tummy muscles pulled in, raise your arm until your elbow is level with your head, and your hand is behind your head, palm facing upward.

2 Extend your arm upward, keeping your elbow close to your head. Keep your tummy muscles tight to keep from straining your back. Slowly lower your arm to the start.

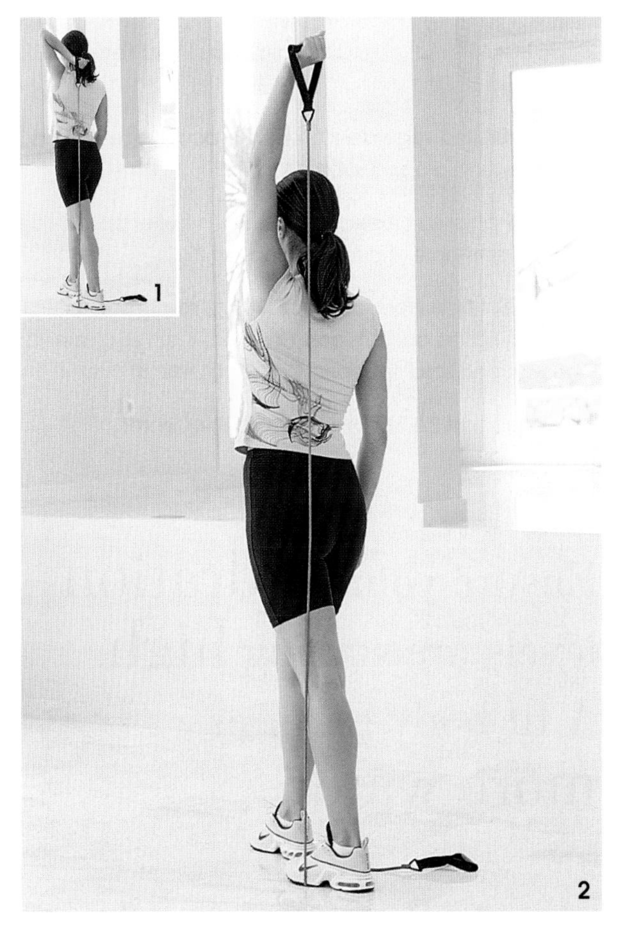

day 42

Your workout today is almost a straight repeat of the previous day's. Make sure your hydration levels are staying high. A fitter body requires more water. You also need more as the workouts become more intense. You should be drinking a minimum of 2½ pints (1.5 liters) a day. Three and a half pints (2 liters) a day is even better. Try not to drink too much when you're eating, though, since this flushes food through your body more quickly and you don't have chance to absorb all the nutrients. Drink most of your water midmorning and midafternoon.

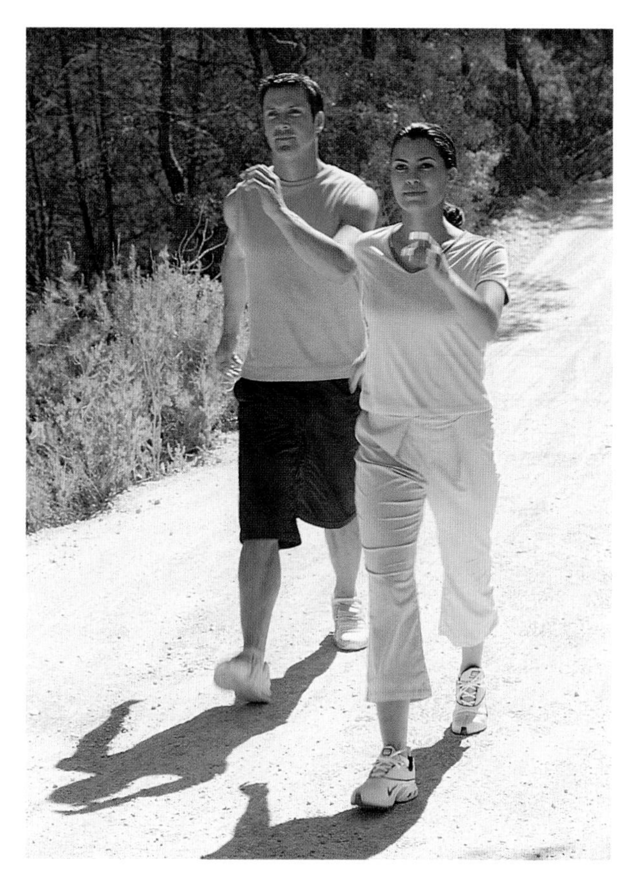

eat&drink

breakfast fresh fruit salad with yogurt and seeds *p132* **or** oatmeal *p132*

lunch broiled vegetable pitas *p139* **or** cottage cheese, cranberry and arugula sandwich *p138*

dinner polenta-crusted swordfish with sweet potato *p145* **or** vegetable and tofu kabobs *p142*

snacks apple, pear, and 4 oz (100 g) raspberries or 1 oz (25 g) dried apricots **and** (for men) 1 oz (25 g) mixed sunflower and sesame seeds, 1 oz (25 g) raisins

drink at least 2½–3½ pints (1.5–2 liters) of water

Ensure your **hydration** levels are staying **high.** A fit body requires **more water.**

three-part workout

Run or fast-pace walk at a constant pace for 30 minutes. Work at 80% MHR (8/10 RPE). This is a slightly higher intensity than your last session, and you'll doubtless find it quite tough because you'll still be feeling some of the effects of yesterday. I have reduced the length of the session, however. As you work, remind yourself of the gains you can make by demanding more and more from yourself.

Move on to repeat the resistance work from day 41. Then, finish the workout with a short standing stretch (*p23*). Like yesterday, take your time over this, so your muscles are good and relaxed at the end of it.

▷ A quick stretch of your leg muscles after a long walk or run will keep stiffness at bay before you do your resistance work. A training buddy will do if there's no wall or rail available to support you as you perform a standing quadricep stretch (*p26*).

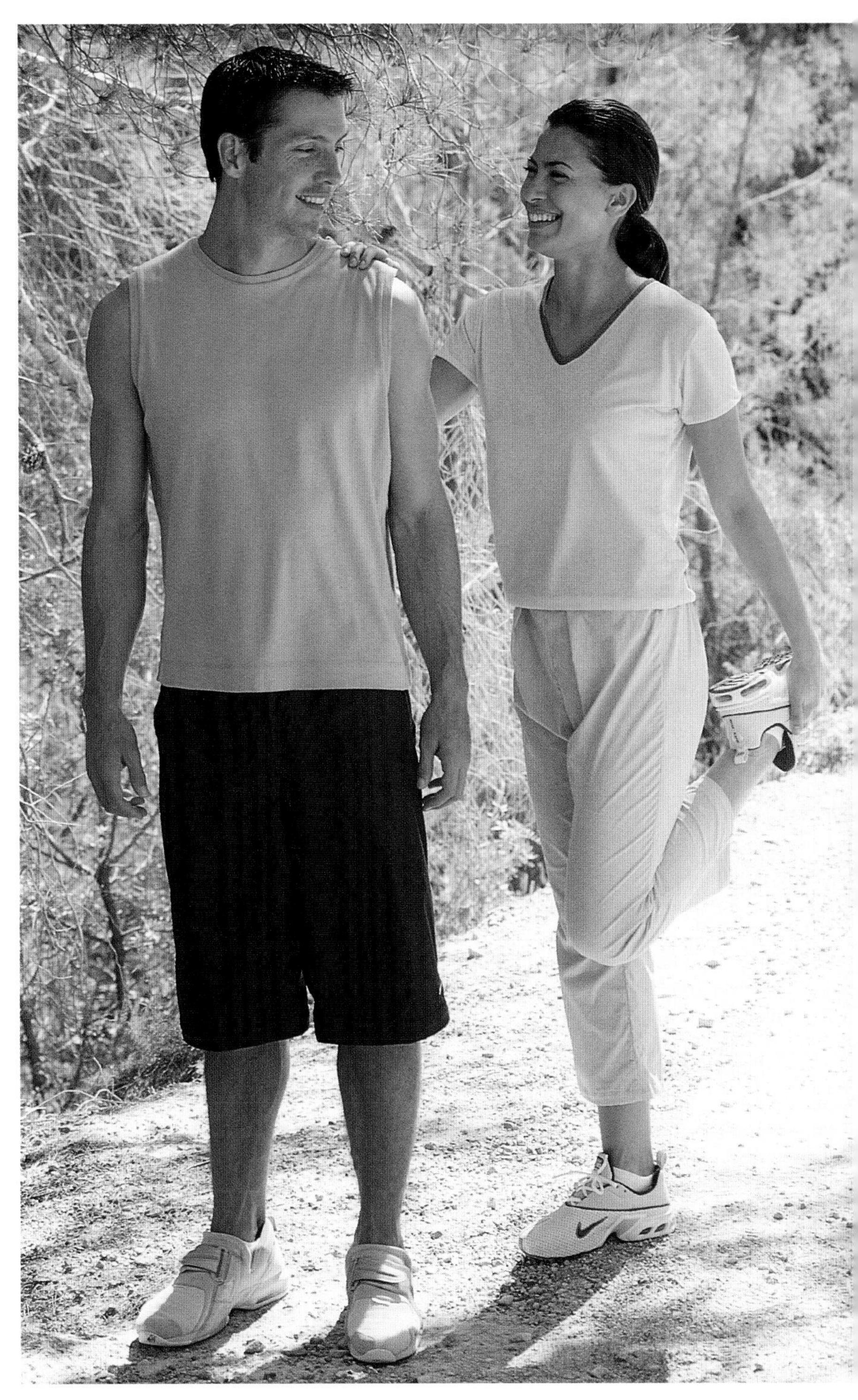

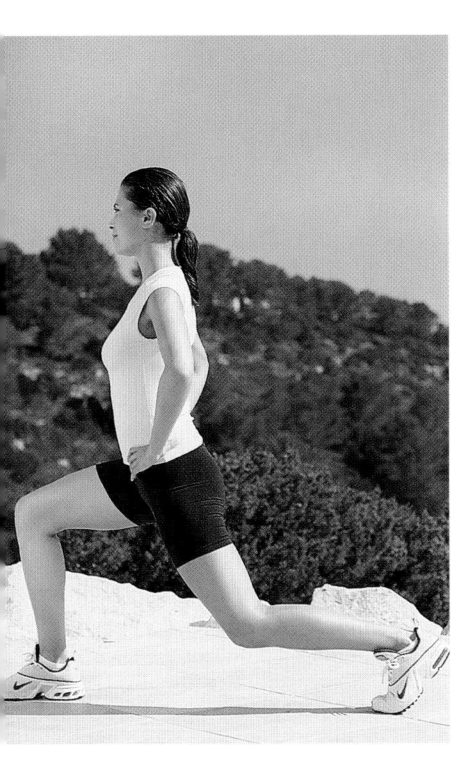

△ In today's resistance, you use PHA, a technique that works your upper and lower body alternately. While the power lunge (*above*) works your legs, the exercises before and after it target your upper arms and shoulders.

week 7

In this penultimate week I always encourage clients to grit their teeth and go for it. If you've drifted away from the plan in any way over the last week, now is the time to create tunnel vision, to blinker yourself from any distractions and outside influences that could keep you from your goal. It's the sprint for the finish...

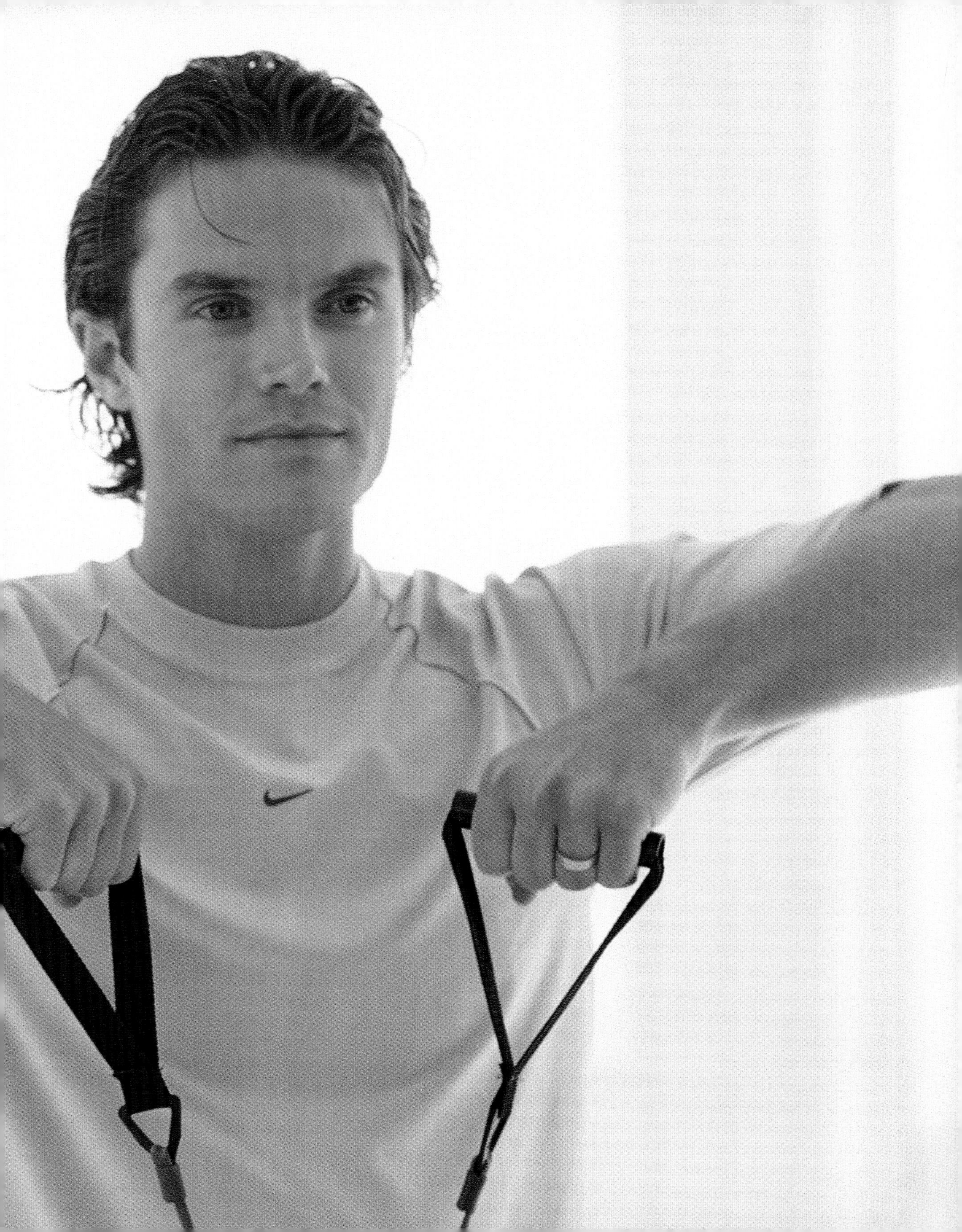

day 43

As the last days tick away, make sure you're doing yourself justice by making the maximum effort you can. Keep yourself mentally strong by repeating your visualization exercise. Picture the body shape you'd like. Superimpose your features on it, then memorize it. Imagine yourself supple, strong, and active. This will be you in two weeks' time.

▽ It's a rest day, but take some time to focus your mind for the final days to come. Lose the distractions in your life. Give yourself the best chance of achieving your goal.

eat&drink

breakfast wheat-free muesli *p132* **or** two slices of whole-wheat toast with nonhydrogenated spread and jam or jelly

lunch asparagus and artichoke salad *p135* **or** green salad *p134*

dinner Thai-style vegetables with polenta *p141* **or** sweet potato gnocchi with tomato and shrimp sauce *p140*

snacks banana, ½ oz (10 g) almonds, 2 oz (50 g) grapes **and** (for men) apple, and 4 oz (100 g) raspberries or 1 oz (25 g) raisins

drink at least 2½–3½ pints (1.5–2 liters) of water

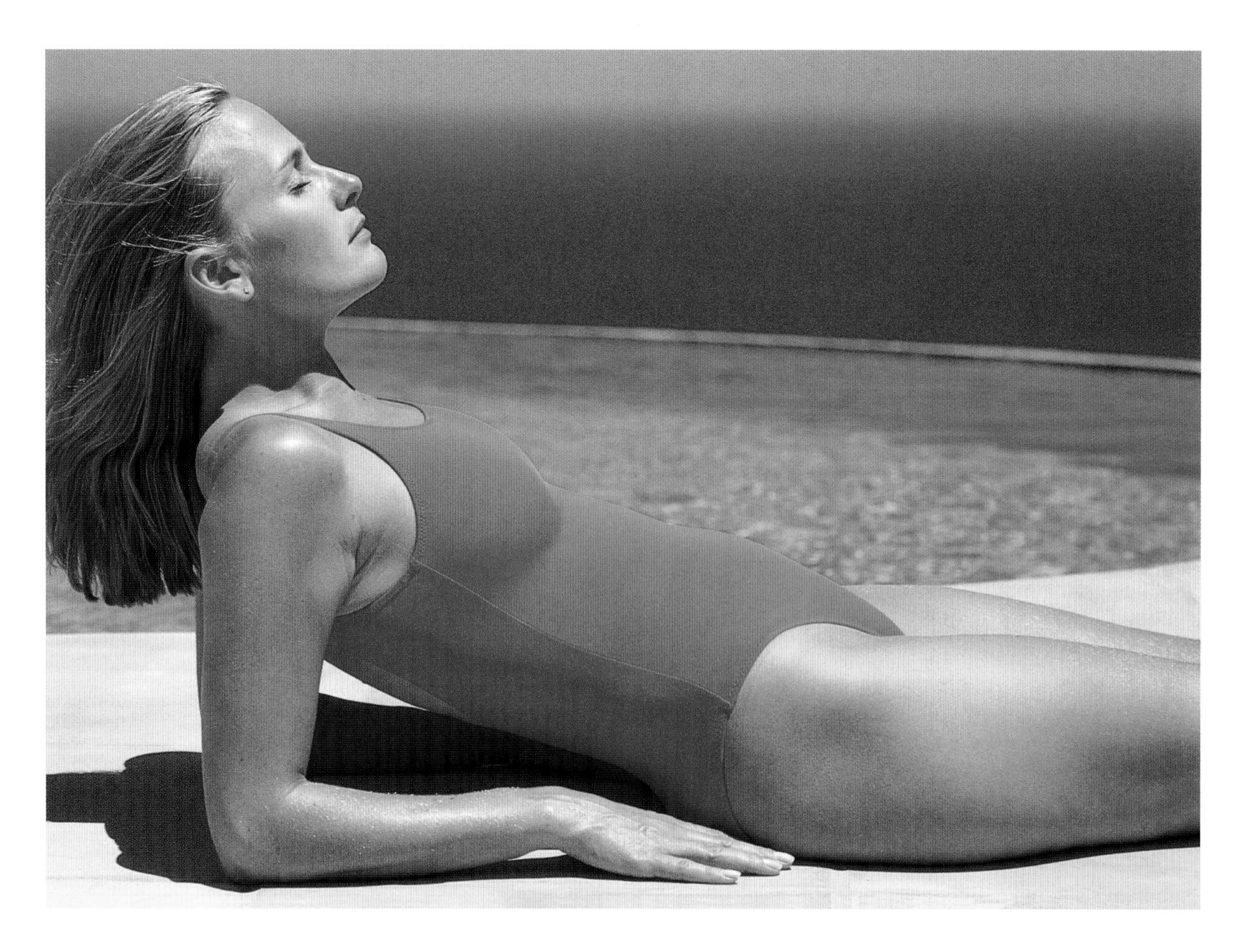

day 44

Back to work, and today, think 'details' – make every part of every workout and every part of what you eat help you attain your desired weight and shape.

eat&drink

breakfast poached egg on two slices of dry whole-wheat toast **or** whole-wheat pancakes *p132*

lunch smoked salmon and dill salad *p138* **or** wild rice salad *p136*

dinner lemon shrimp with three bean salad *p148* **or** Asian stir fry *p141*

snacks apple, pear, 1 oz (25 g) sunflower seeds, 1 oz (25 g) raisins **and** (for men) banana, 1 oz (25 g) sunflower seeds, ½ oz (10 g) raisins

drink at least 2½–3½ pints (1.5–2 liters) of water

three-part workout

1 cardio

Fast-pace walk for 2 minutes, then run for 3 minutes. Repeat this five times so you walk and run a total of six times. Run at 85% MHR (8–9/10 RPE).

2 resistance

The exercises today are super sets. Do the first six in order, with 10-second rests in between exercises. Rest for 1 minute, then repeat the sequence three times, with 1-minute rests between complete sets. Do the next five in the same way, but repeat them only once, with a 1-minute rest between sets.

3 stretching

Finish the workout with a total body stretch (*p22*).

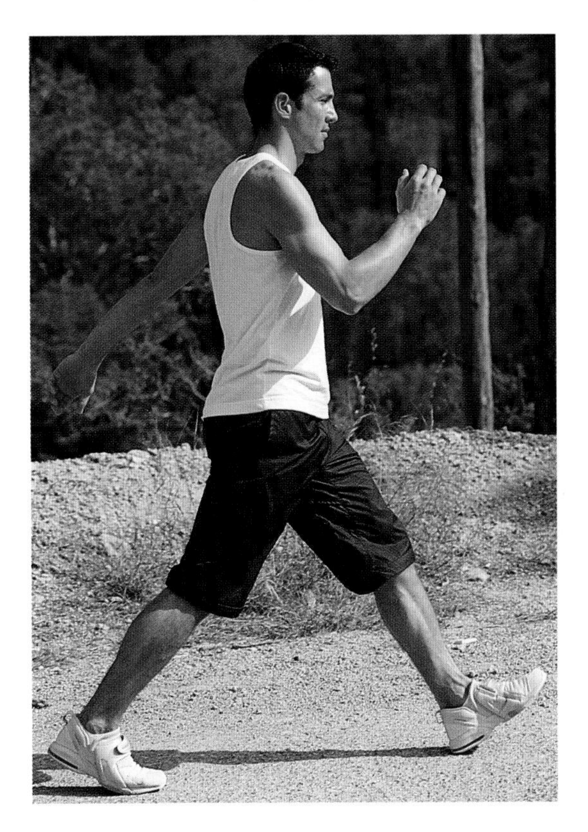

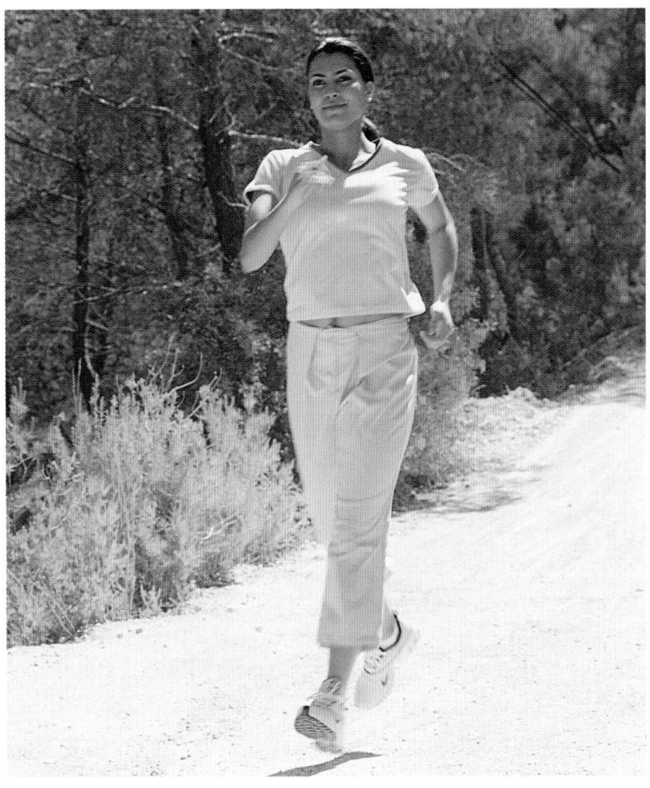

day 44 resistance work

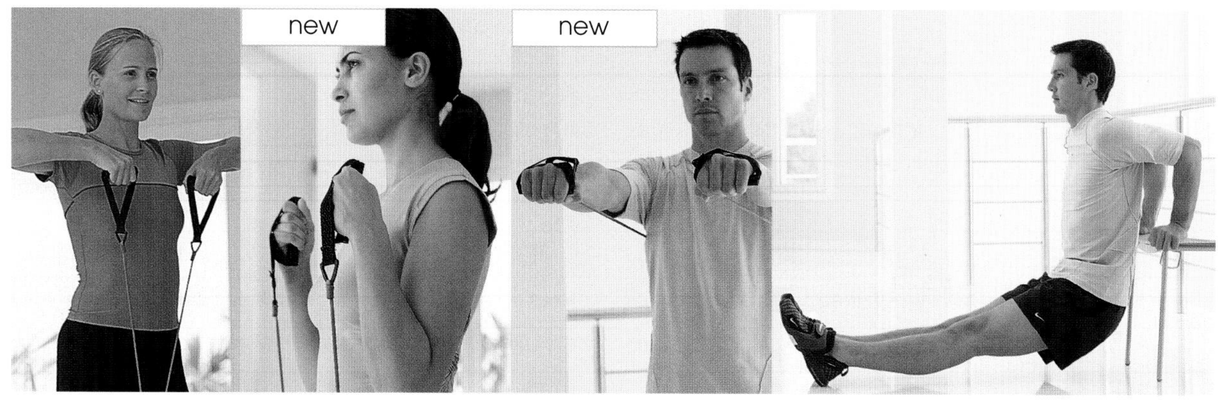

upright row *p62*
① 15 reps ② 20 reps

hammer curl *p111*
① 15 reps ② 15 reps

chest press *p111*
① 15 reps ② 15 reps

advanced dip *p98*
① 20 reps ② 25 reps

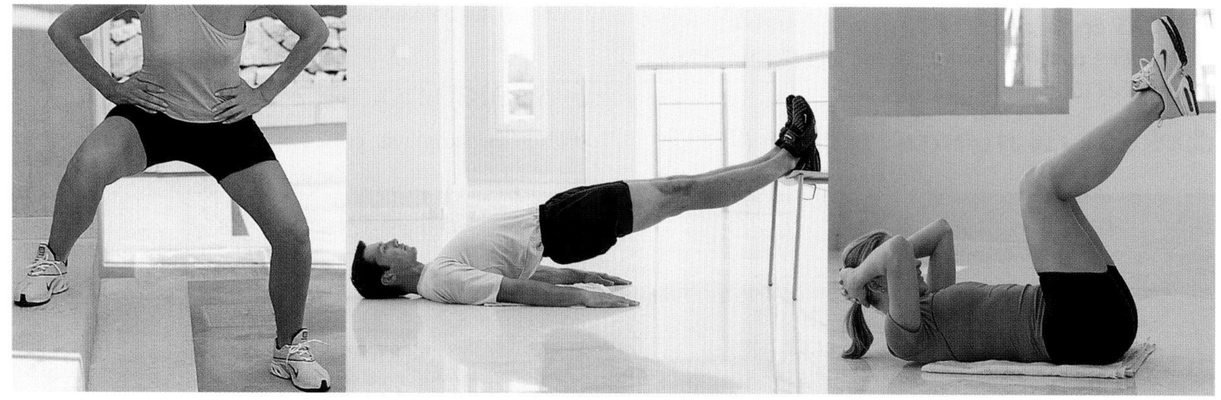

step squat *p87*
① 12 per leg ② 15 per leg

glute bridge *p87*
① 30 secs ② 30 secs x4

full crunch *p68*
① 20 reps ② 30 reps

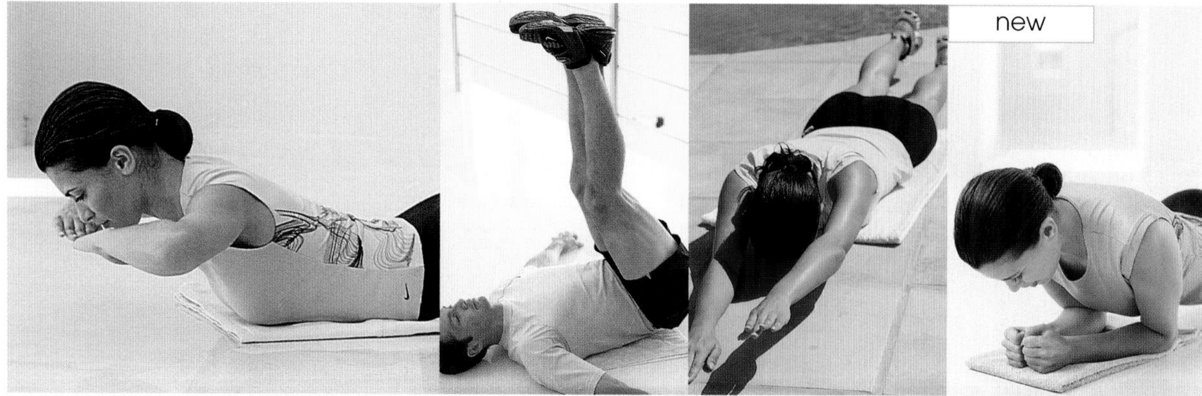

back extension *p38*
① 20 reps ② 25 reps

reverse curl *p43*
① 20 reps ② 25 reps

dorsal raise *p92*
① & ② 20 reps per side

bridge *p111*
① 30 secs ② 30 secs x2

day 44 new exercises

hammer curl ▷

A variation on the bicep curl, the hammer curl targets the outer side of your upper arms, making them look longer and leaner.

1 Stand with your feet hip-width apart in the middle of the exertube, knees slightly bent. Hold a handle of the exertube in each hand, palms facing inward. Keep your back straight and your tummy muscles pulled in.

2 Lift the handles toward your shoulders, keeping your elbows tucked in. With knuckles facing each other, flex your biceps at the top of the movement. Don't allow your body to sway. Slowly lower your arms to the start position.

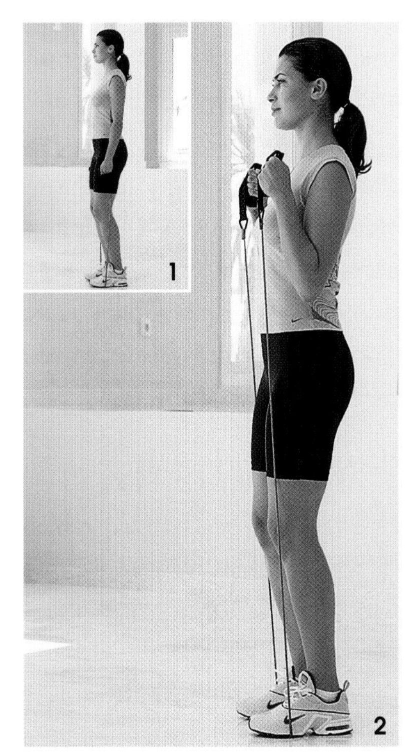

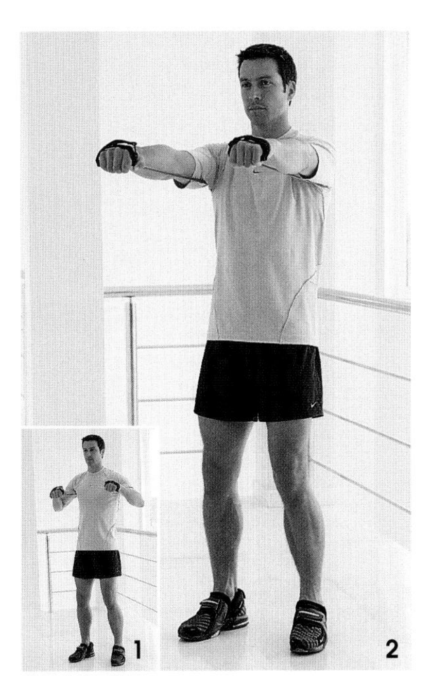

chest press ◁

Very effective at working the muscles of your chest and the backs of your upper arms.

1 Stand with your legs hip-width apart, knees slightly bent. Keep your back straight and your tummy muscles pulled in. Wrap the exertube cord once around each hand, then place it around your back and under your arms. Push your elbows out to the sides, with your hands just in front of your chest and your palms facing downward.

2 Extend your arms out in front of you, palms facing down. Keep your back straight and your shoulder blades back. Slowly pull your arms back to the start.

bridge ▷

This gives great tone to your tummy. What's more, you don't need to move a muscle! Just hold it still.

Position yourself with your toes on the floor and your elbows directly below your shoulders. Keeping a straight line from your shoulders to your ankles, raise yourself up so your elbows and toes support your body. Use your tummy muscles to maintain the position. Slowly return to the start.

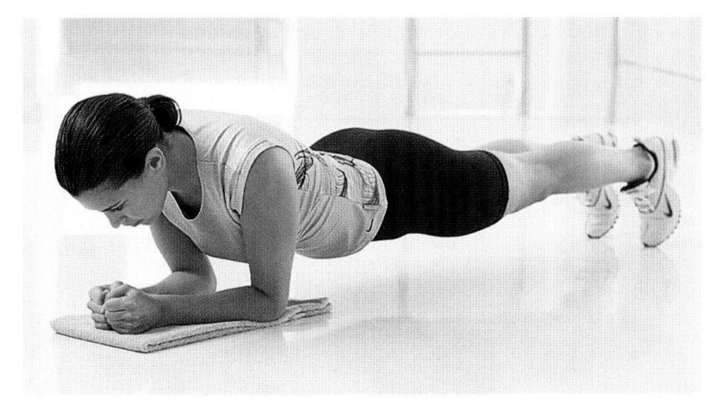

day 45

The end is now in sight. If, by any chance, you do find yourself starting to falter at this point, call upon the help of the person you've chosen as your support network. After advising you for the past few weeks, they're bound to feel almost a personal stake in your achievement. Bounce any problems off them. Ask them to help you stay focused on your goals. You never know when you may be asked to do the same for them.

eat & drink

breakfast fresh fruit salad with yogurt and seeds *p132* **or** raspberry fool *p132*

lunch broiled vegetable pitas *p139* **or** cottage cheese, cranberry and arugula sandwich *p138*

dinner monkfish with roasted vegetables *p146* **or** mushroom risotto *p142*

snacks apple, pear, and 4 oz (100 g) raspberries or 1 oz (25 g) dried apricots **and** (for men) 1 oz (25 g) mixed sunflower and sesame seeds, 1 oz (25 g) raisins

drink at least 2½–3½ pints (1.5–2 liters) of water

If you can't see the forest for the trees, think of the positive changes you've made. You're well on the road to success.

day 46

Your resistance work for today is a repeat of the program from day 44. Like then, your cardio work is interval training, but for this session I've increased the intensity a little. I've also reduced the length of the intervals.

eat & drink

breakfast wheat-free muesli *p132* **or** oatmeal *p132*

lunch smoked salmon and dill salad *p138* **or** wild rice salad *p136*

dinner broiled or steamed fish with quinoa *p143* **or** chicken with couscous and mint yogurt *p149*

snacks banana, ½ oz (10 g) almonds, 2 oz (50 g) grapes **and** (for men) apple, and 4 oz (100 g) raspberries or 1 oz (25 g) raisins

drink at least 2½–3½ pints (1.5–2 liters) of water

three-part workout

For your cardio work today, there's more interval training. Fast-pace walk for 1 minute, then run for 2 minutes. Repeat this five times, so you walk and run a total of six times. Run at 85–90% MHR (8–9/10 RPE). Move on to repeat the resistance program from day 44. Then finish the workout with a total body stretch (*p22*).

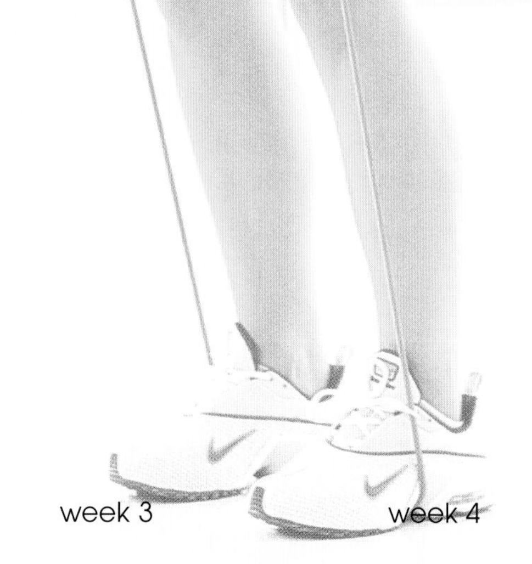

day 47

Before you started the fat loss plan, you had to assess how fit and healthy you were. In the questionnaire on page 14, I asked you how often you ate dinner after 8 o'clock in the evening. You may have wondered why. Well, the fact is that the later you have your dinner, the harder it is for your body to digest it.

There are always going to be times when you can't eat before 8 o'clock, however. The solution is to have more alkaline and vegetable-based meals at that time of the evening. This is already taken care of for you while you're on the fat loss plan, but for guidance in the future, take another look at pages 30–31 for a list of foods that fit the bill.

eat&drink

breakfast poached egg on two slices of dry whole-wheat toast **or** whole-wheat pancakes *p132*

lunch salade niçoise *p137* **or** Greek salad *p134*

dinner broiled fish with sweet potato and spinach bake *p144* **or** marinated chicken with steamed vegetables *p149*

snacks apple, pear, 1 oz (25 g) sunflower seeds, 1 oz (25 g) raisins **and** (for men) banana, 1 oz (25 g) sunflower seeds, ½ oz (10 g) raisins

drink at least 2½–3½ pints (1.5–2 liters) of water

▽ The fat loss plan dinners are relatively light meals of vegetables and protein. Even so, do your best to eat before 8 o'clock in the evening – that gives your body plenty of time to digest the food before you go to bed.

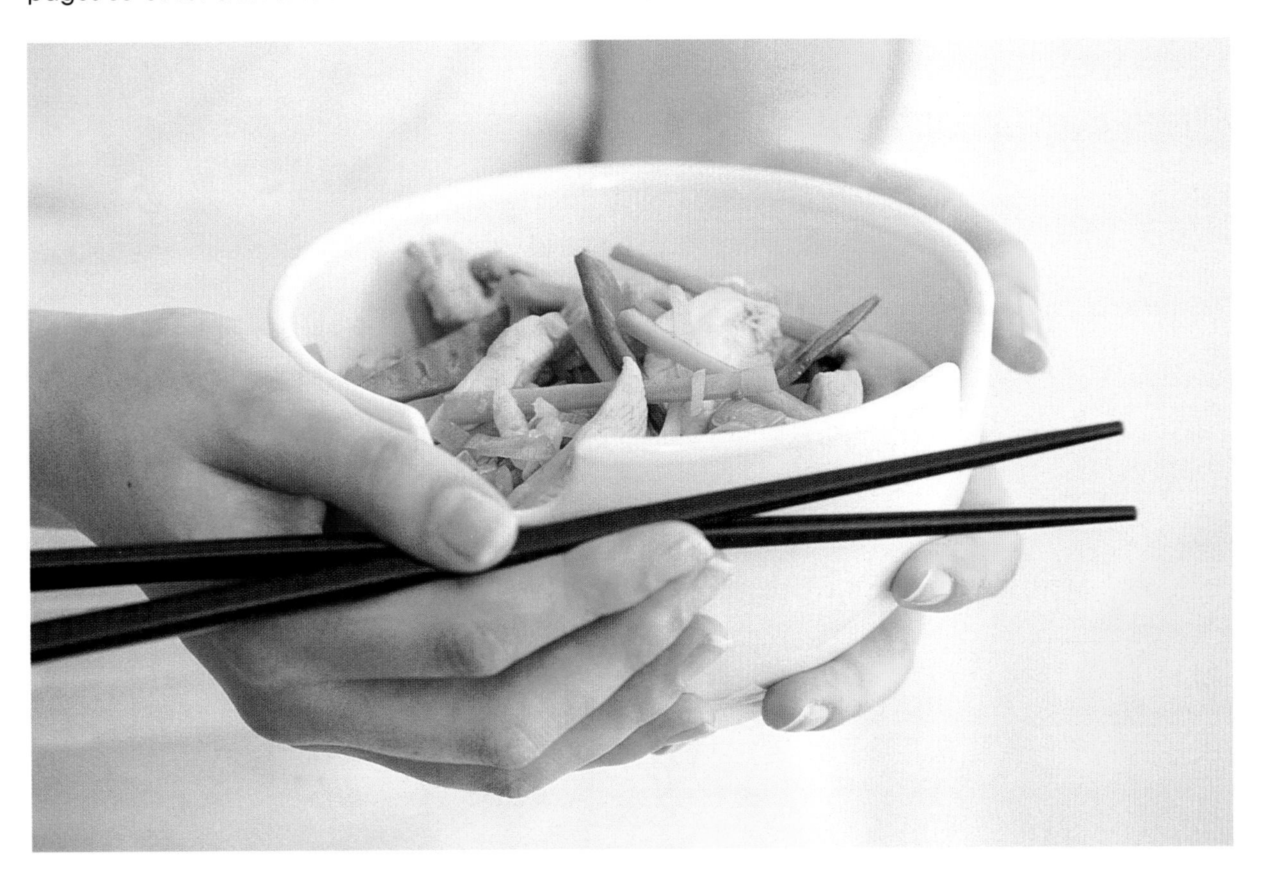

day 48

This is another 'cardio only' day, and it's a big 'cardio only' day – a 60-minute session. This may seem like a long time to run or fast-pace walk, and I bet you wouldn't have contemplated it seven weeks ago. Now, you're about to do it, and it even seems perfectly normal.

Push yourself as hard as you can through the session. Keep checking your heart rate – you're so much fitter now, and what made you work hard before is not what makes you work hard these days. Increase your level in line with your heart-rate target. Your legs may get tired and your arms may feel stiff, but you're giving yourself the best possible chance to achieve your goal next week.

eat&drink

breakfast fresh fruit salad with yogurt and seeds *p132* **or** oatmeal *p132*

lunch broccoli salad *p135* **or** beet and carrot salad *p134*

dinner marinated chicken with steamed vegetables *p149* **or** wheat-free pasta with turkey *p148*

snacks apple, pear, and 4 oz (100 g) raspberries or 1 oz (25 g) dried apricots **and** (for men) 1 oz (25 g) mixed sunflower and sesame seeds, 1 oz (25 g) raisins

drink at least 2½–3½ pints (1.5–2 liters) of water

two-part workout

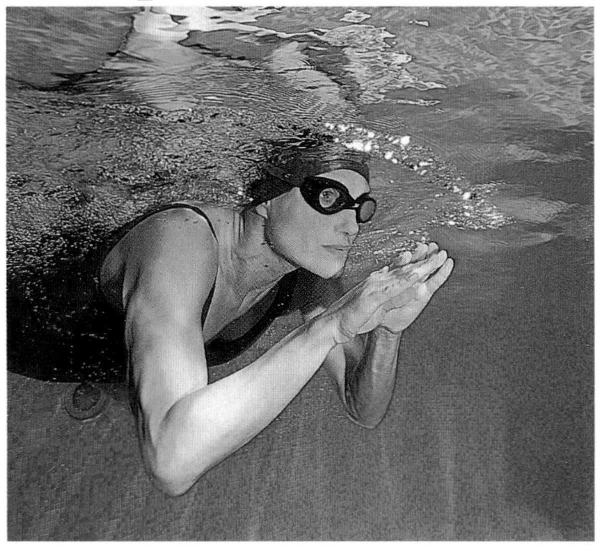

1 cardio

Run or fast-pace walk at a constant pace for 60 minutes. Work at 70% MHR (7/10 RPE).

For a long cardio session like this, it's best to plan your route carefully before you set out. Aim to make it as interesting – and as challenging for your body – as possible. A larger circuit, where you venture far afield, is great if the weather's good. But it pays to be confident that you'll be back at home when your 60 minutes are up – you may surprise yourself by how much ground you can cover in an hour. If you're in any doubt about this, choose a shorter route and do several circuits.

Keeping your hydration levels high is of the utmost importance, too. So, make sure you take plenty of water along with you, particularly if the weather is hot.

2 stretching

Finish the workout with a short standing stretch (*p23*). Linger over each of the stretches if you can spare the time – your muscles may find the long cardio session rather punishing.

day 49

Both the cardio and resistance parts of today's workout will test your cardiovascular system enormously. They'll also burn lots of calories.

eat&drink

breakfast wheat-free muesli *p132* **or** two slices of whole-wheat toast with nonhydrogenated spread and jam or jelly

lunch asparagus and artichoke salad *p135* **or** Camargue rice salad *p136*

dinner Thai-style vegetables with polenta *p141* **or** carrot and sweet potato fishcakes with herb salad *p144*

snacks banana, ½ oz (10 g) almonds, 2 oz (50 g) grapes **and** (for men) apple, and 4 oz (100 g) raspberries or 1 oz (25 g) raisins

drink at least 2½–3½ pints (1.5–2 liters) of water

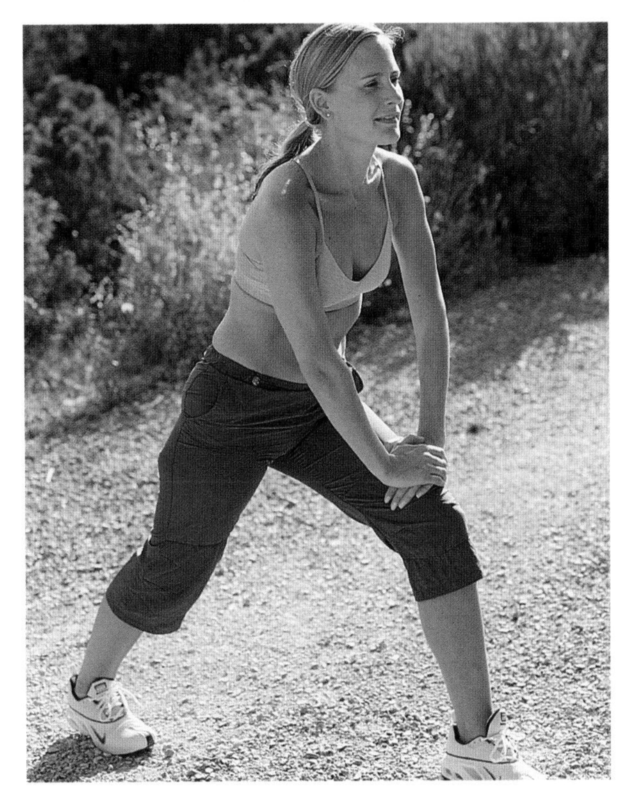

three-part workout

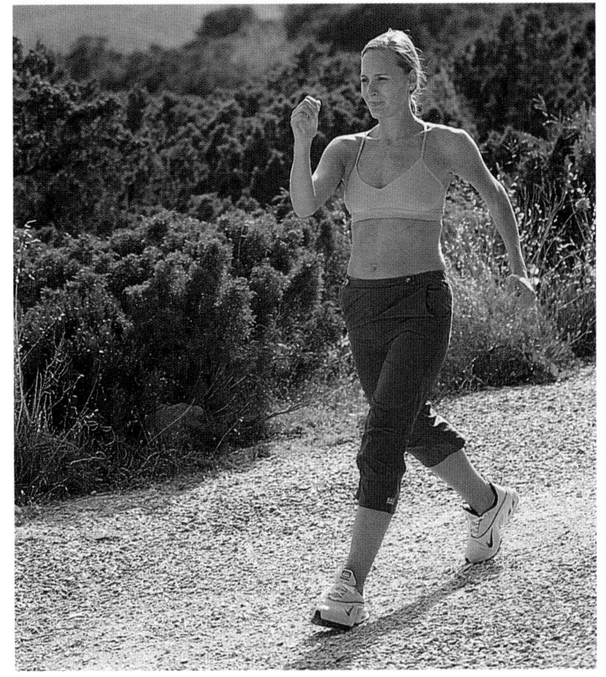

1 cardio

If you ran on day 48, then fast-pace walk today (or vice versa). Fast-pace walk or run at a constant pace for 30 minutes. Work at 75% MHR (7–8/10 RPE).

2 resistance

The resistance for today is based on PHA. Do the reps for the exercises in order, resting for 15 seconds between each one. After the oblique crunch, rest for 2 minutes, and then repeat the sequence. Level ② users, make sure you have plenty of resistance on your exertube (*see day 9*).

3 stretching

End the workout with a total body stretch (*p22*).

◁ At this point in the plan, spend 5–10 minutes a day doing general stretching. A calf stretch (*p27*) is particularly good after a run or walk. Don't stretch excessively, though, since this won't increase your flexibility.

day 49 resistance work

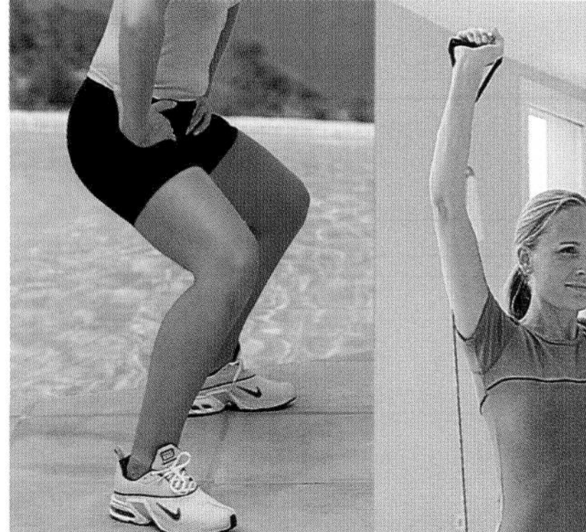

wide squat *p52*
① 20 reps ② 30 reps

shoulder press *p52*
① 20 reps ② 12 reps

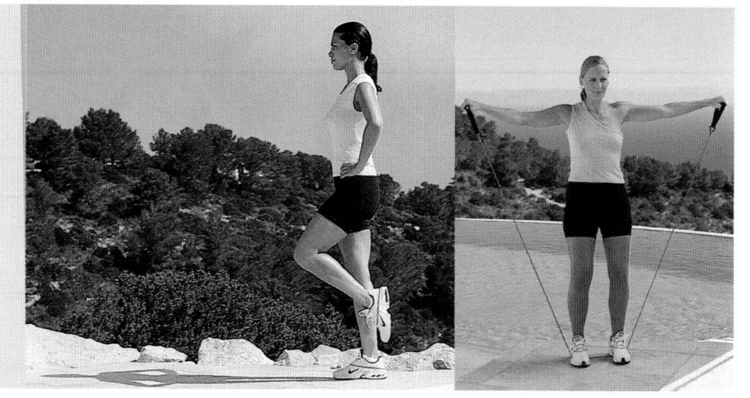

walking lunge *p75*
① 20 strides ② 20 strides

lateral raise *p21*
① 20 reps ② 12 reps

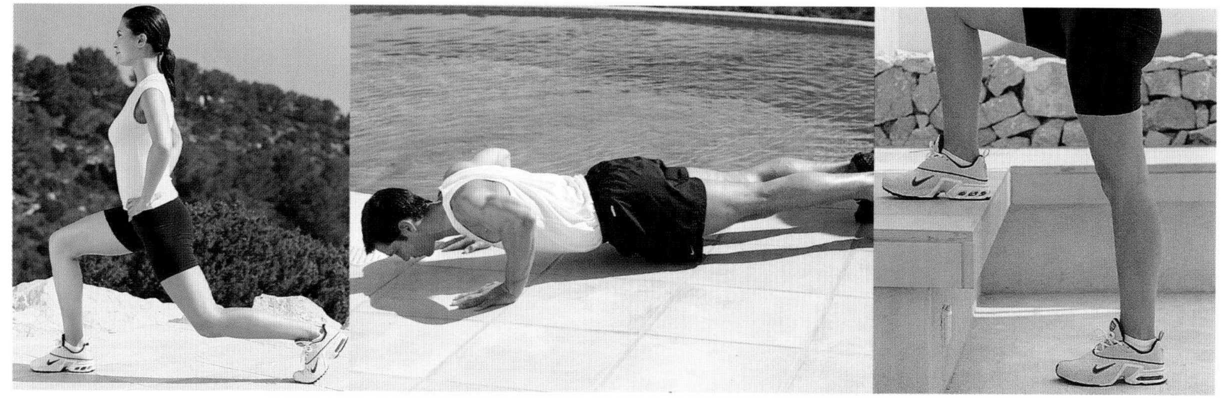

power lunge *p75*
① 15 per leg ② 20 per leg

push-up *p98*
① 10 reps ② 15 reps

step-up *p62*
① 15 reps per leg ② 20 reps per leg

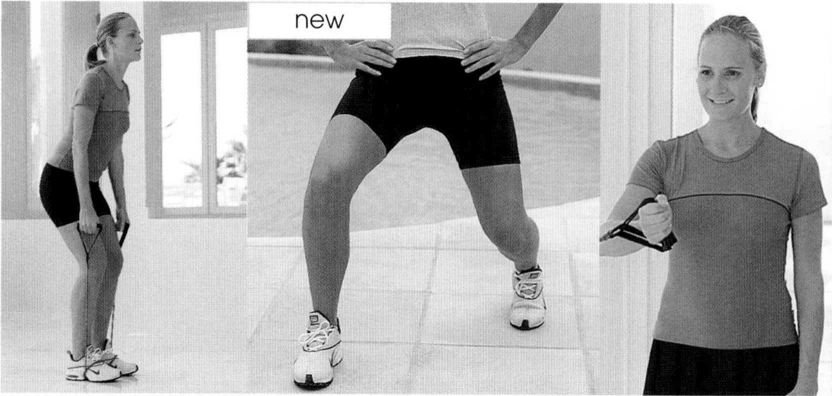

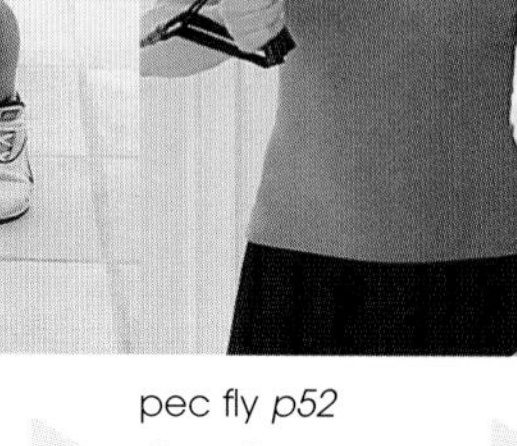

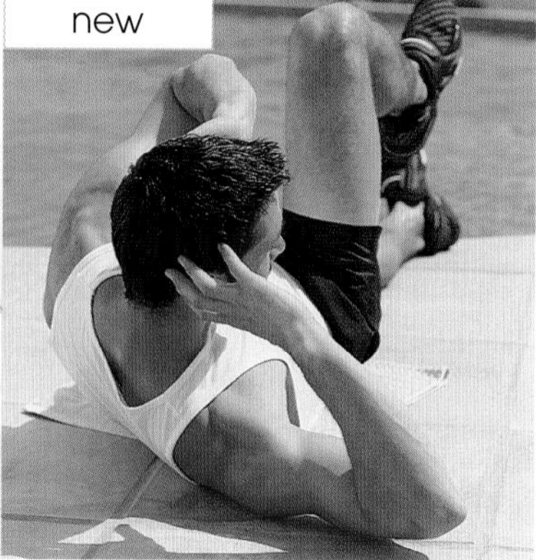

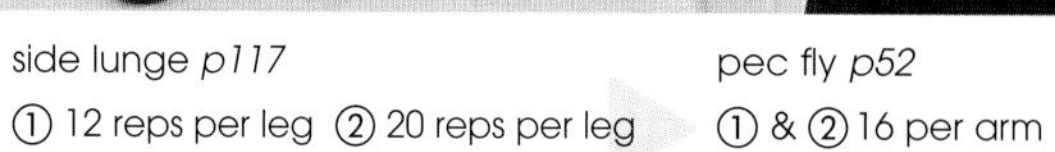

upright row *p62*
① 15 reps ② 12 reps

side lunge *p117*
① 12 reps per leg ② 20 reps per leg

pec fly *p52*
① & ② 16 per arm

oblique crunch *p117*
①15 reps per side ② 25 reps per side x2

day 49 new exercises

side lunge ▷

This variation on the 'basic' lunge uses more of the muscles around your hips and bottom. It makes your inner thighs work harder, too.

1 Stand with your feet hip-width apart, knees slightly bent. Place your hands on your hips.

2 Take a step forward diagonally at 45° and plant your foot about one stride-length from your back foot. Keep your hips facing forward, your body upright, and your tummy muscles pulled in. Bend your knees to bring your front knee directly over your front foot, but don't allow it to go farther forward than the laces of your shoe. Lower your back knee until it's about 6 in (15 cm) off the floor. Put your weight on the heel of your front foot to work the muscles of your buttock. Slowly return to the start position.

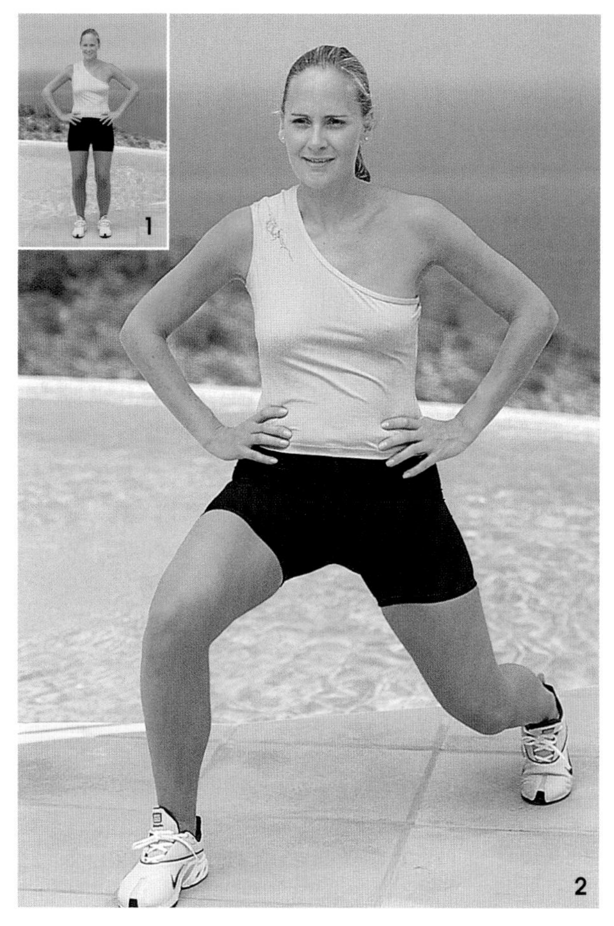

oblique crunch ▷

For those of you who have 'handles' rather than obliques! (Your obliques are the muscles at the side of your tummy.)

1 Lie on your back with one knee bent and the other leg flat on the floor. Place your hands by your ears.

2 Slowly raise your opposite shoulder and elbow up toward the outside of your raised thigh. Lower your shoulder and leg to the start position slowly.

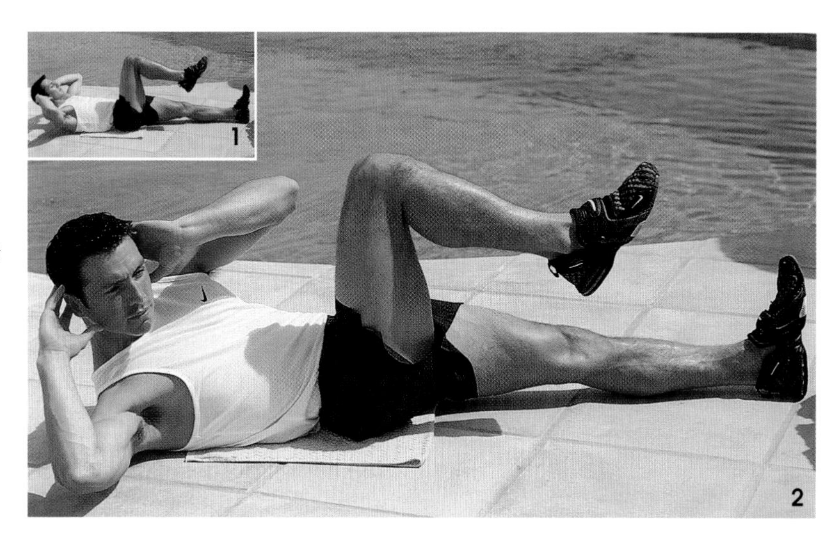

week 8

This is going to be a quality and quantity week. The technical term for what you're about to do is 'drying out your muscles' – which means making them look as lean and toned as possible. You'll do it with high reps and short recovery periods. Your fat will keep burning away, but you won't be building muscle, you'll be sculpting it.

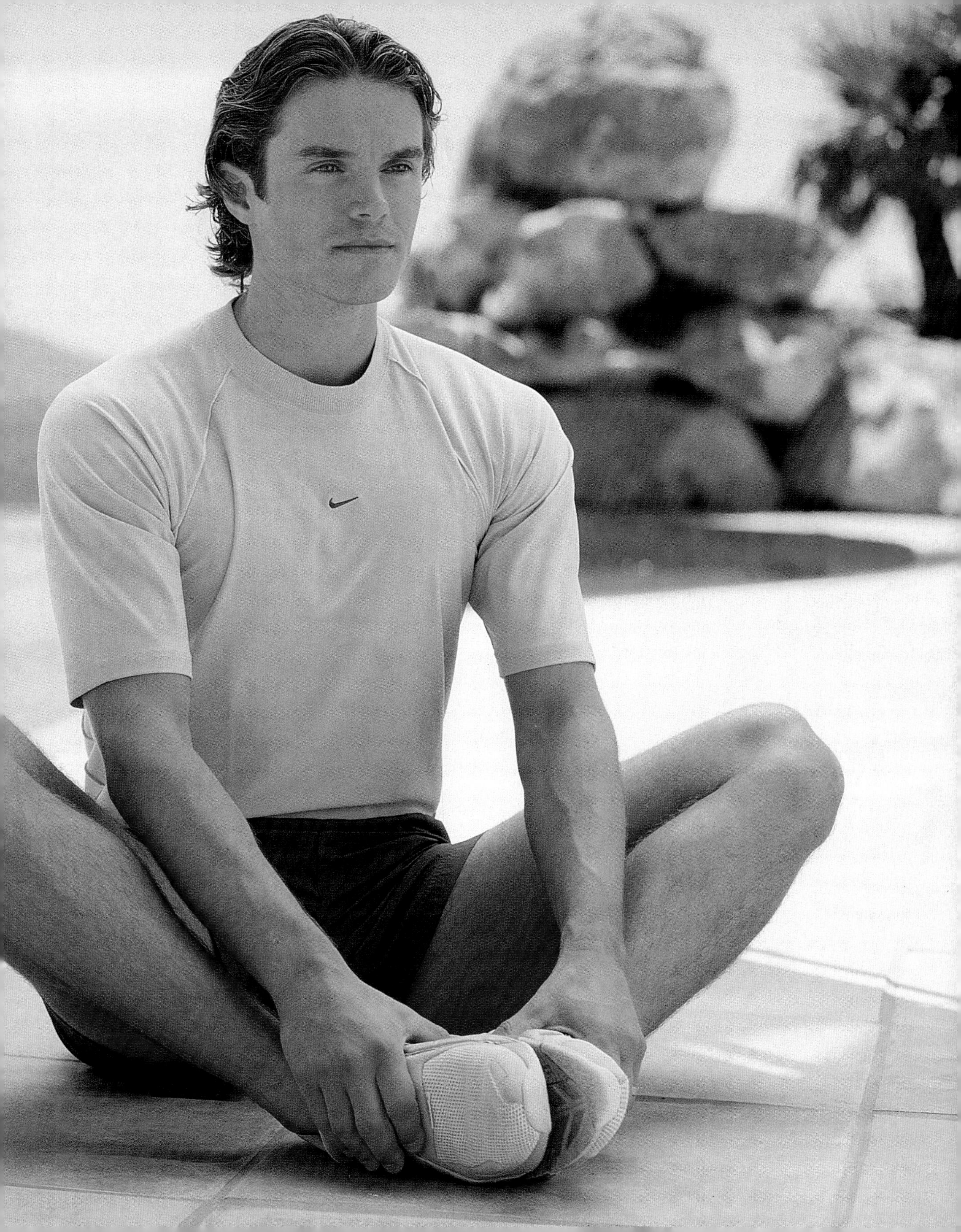

day 50

This is the final week of the plan, and that means absolute focus is required of you. To make sure you feel great by day 56, I don't want you to put a foot wrong. Think of yourself as a singer signed to record a video at the end of the week, or an athlete preparing for an important race. You want to look and be your best. You've been building toward this for seven weeks, so make the most of the big final push. Starting today.

eat&drink

breakfast poached egg on two slices of dry whole-wheat toast **or** whole-wheat pancakes *p132*

lunch salade niçoise *p137* **or** Greek salad *p134*

dinner smoked salmon and lentil salad *p147* **or** vegetable and tofu kabobs *p142*

snacks apple, pear, 1 oz (25 g) sunflower seeds, 1 oz (25 g) raisins **and** (for men) banana, 1 oz (25 g) sunflower seeds, ½ oz (10 g) raisins

drink at least 2½–3½ pints (1.5–2 liters) of water

Remember that promise to yourself seven weeks ago? You're pushing to fit into those jeans.

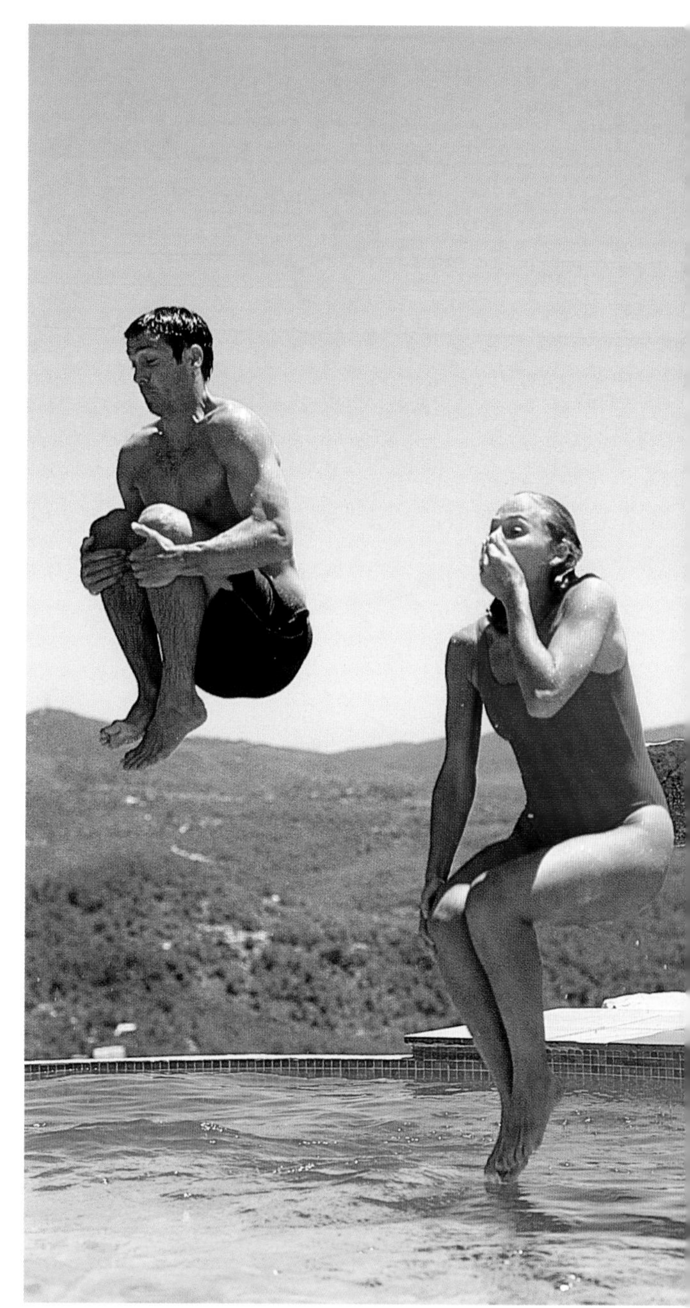

△ You can't quite celebrate just yet, but you're bound to be feeling a sense of relief that you've almost made it to the end. Don't let worries about the future cloud your sense of jubilation – I'll let you know what to do. In the meantime, keep focused.

day 51

Today you'll begin the 'drying out' process on your muscles, stripping away the buildup of excess fluid in them so they look lean and toned. High reps mean the blood will be pumping to all parts of your body, and your muscles will be working intensively. Instead of building muscle, you'll be sculpting it.

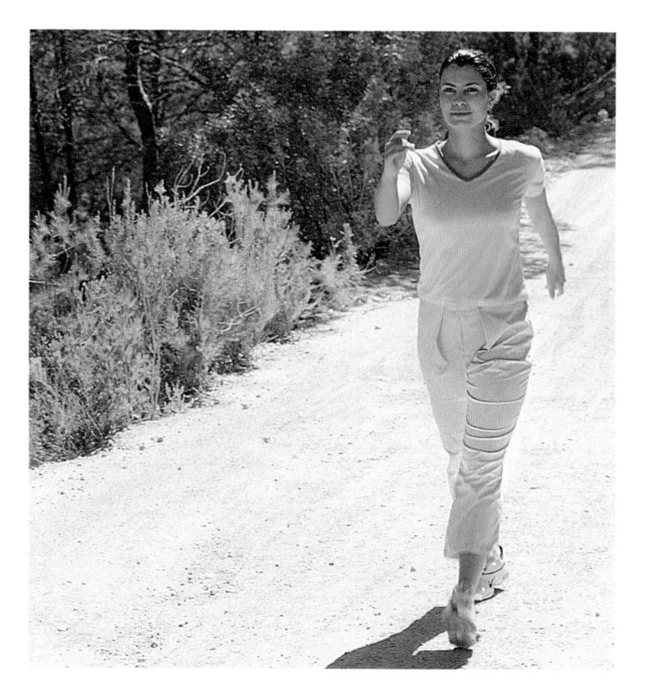

eat&drink

breakfast fresh fruit salad with yogurt and seeds *p132* **or** raspberry fool *p132*

lunch broiled vegetable pitas *p139* **or** cottage cheese, cranberry and arugula sandwich *p138*

dinner monkfish with roasted vegetables *p146* **or** mushroom risotto *p142*

snacks apple, pear, and 4 oz (100 g) raspberries or 1 oz (25 g) dried apricots **and** (for men) 1 oz (25 g) mixed sunflower and sesame seeds, 1 oz (25 g) raisins

drink at least 2½–3½ pints (1.5–2 liters) of water

three-part workout

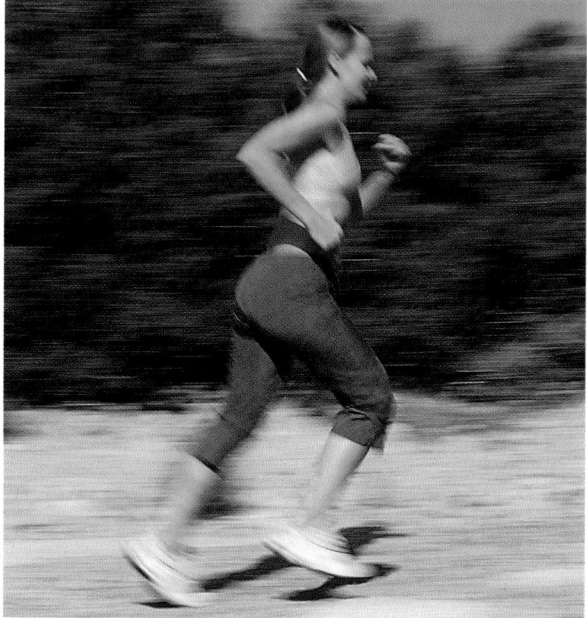

1 cardio

Today, you'll be doing interval training. Fast-pace walk for 1 minute, then run for 2 minutes. Repeat this nine times, so you walk and run a total of 10 times. Run at 85–90% MHR (8–9/10 RPE).

2 resistance

The resistance work for today is super sets. Perform the first four exercises in order, repeat the entire sequence, and then rest for 1 minute. Perform the next four exercises in order, repeat the whole sequence, and then rest for 1 minute. Perform the last four exercises in order, and then repeat them, too.

3 stretching

End today's workout with a total body stretch (*p22*). If you have the time, linger over each stretch move so you relax your muscles thoroughly. And keep pushing the stretches, so you maintain improvement.

day 51 resistance work

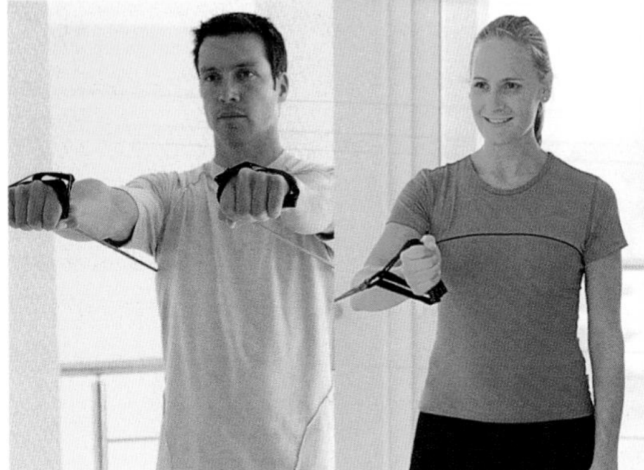

chest press *p111*
① & ② 12 reps

pec flye *p52*
① & ② 12 reps per arm

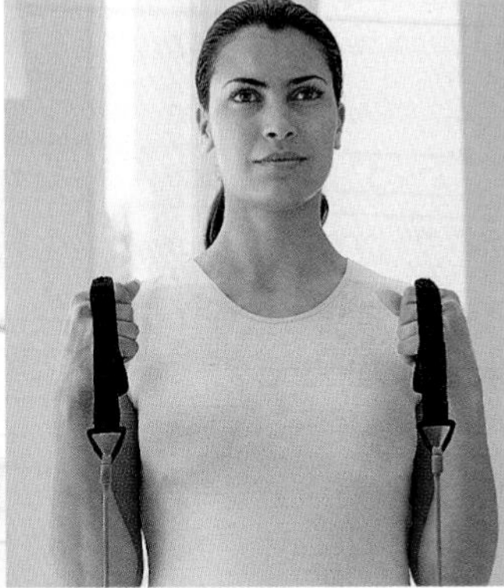

hammer curl *p111*
① 12 reps ② 12 reps

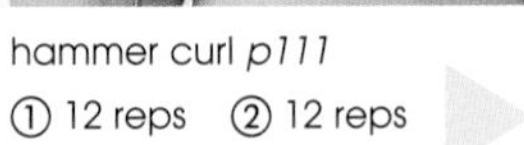

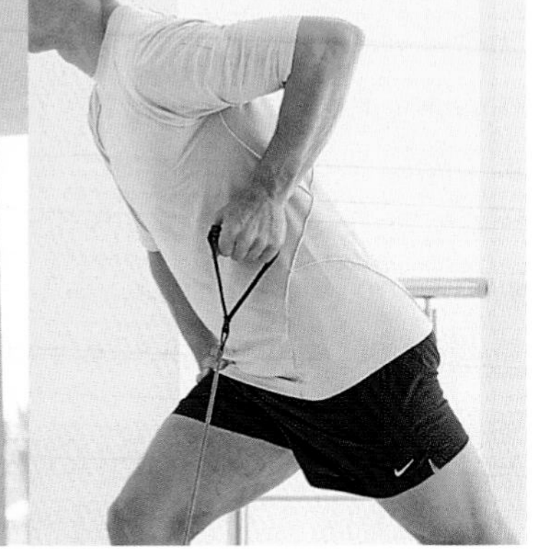

single-arm row *p68*
① & ② 12 reps per arm x2

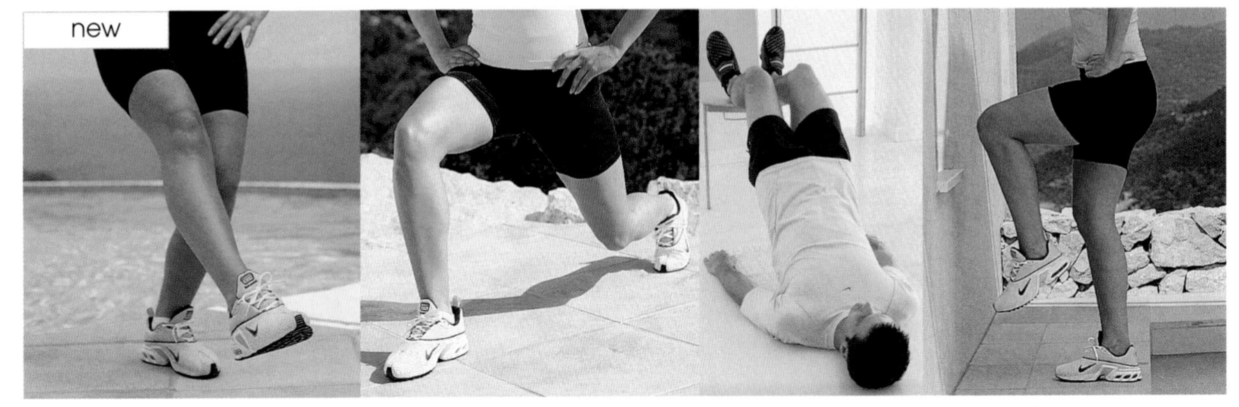

single-leg squat *p123*
① 12 per leg ② 15 per leg

power lunge *p75*
① 15 per leg ② 20 per leg

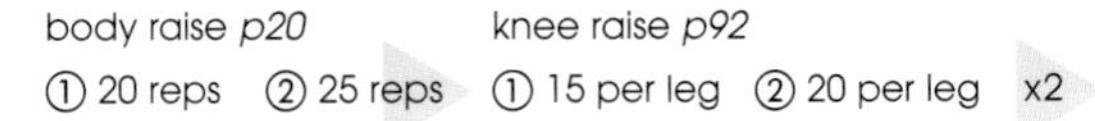

body raise *p20*
① 20 reps ② 25 reps

knee raise *p92*
① 15 per leg ② 20 per leg x2

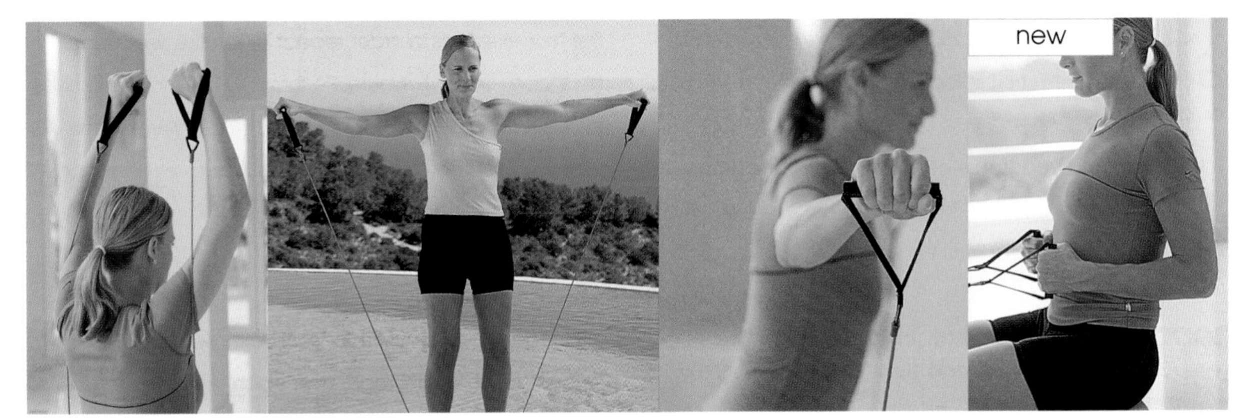

shoulder press *p52*
① 12 reps ② 25 reps

lateral raise *p21*
① 12 reps ② 20 reps

bent-over lateral raise *p87*
① 15 reps ② 20 reps

seated row *p123*
① 12 reps ② 20 reps x2

day 51 new exercises

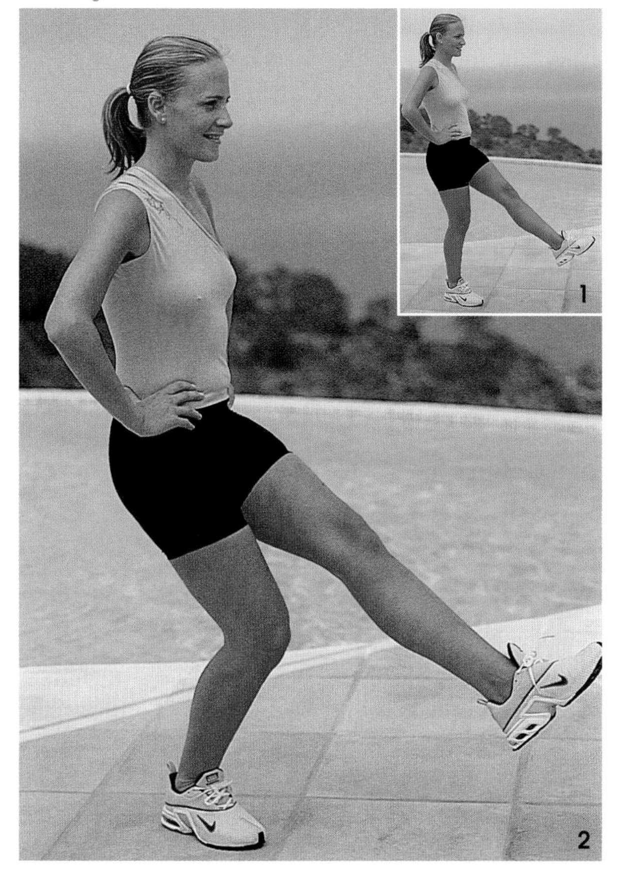

single-leg squat ◁

You may find this exercise a little tricky to begin with, but once you've mastered the balancing act, you'll see speedy results in your bottom and thighs.

1 Stand with your feet hip-width apart, knees slightly bent. Place your hands on your hips. Keep your back straight and your tummy muscles pulled in. Raise one leg in front of you, keeping it straight ahead of you, with your heel about 6 in (15 cm) off the floor.

2 Imagining you're about to sit on a chair, lower yourself down, keeping your back straight as you do so. Control the movement with your supporting leg – it should never be allowed to bend to less than 90° at the back of the knee. Slowly raise yourself to the start position.

seated row ▷

An exercise that makes your upper arms work hard. Squeeze your shoulder blades together as you perform it so you maximize the work in your upper back muscles, too.

1 Wrap the exertube around a stationary pole or handle at about shin height. Sit slightly farther than leg-length from the pole, with your legs stretched out in front of you. Hold the handles of the exertube with palms facing each other. Keep your back straight and your tummy pulled in.

2 Pull the exertube handles toward you. Aim for the lower chest/tummy area and squeeze your elbows close to your body. Slowly return to the start position.

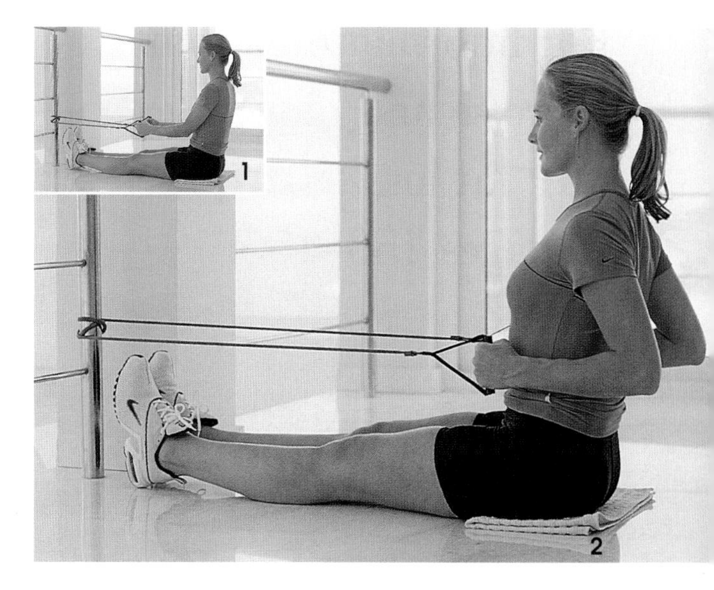

day 52

You're almost at the end of the plan and starting to feel a bit concerned, perhaps, about what the next step will be. Try not to worry about that now – in the 'going forward' section on pages 150–155, I reveal all about keeping yourself lean and fit, from the kind of exercise you should do to the type of food you should eat. For the moment, though, enjoy the rest of this week and allow yourself to feel good about your accomplishments.

eat & drink

breakfast wheat-free muesli *p132* **or** oatmeal *p132*

lunch smoked salmon and dill salad *p138* **or** wild rice salad *p136*

dinner broiled or steamed fish with quinoa *p143* **or** chicken with couscous and mint yogurt *p149*

snacks banana, ½ oz (10 g) almonds, 2 oz (50 g) grapes **and** (for men) apple, and 4 oz (100 g) raspberries or 1 oz (25 g) raisins

drink at least 2½–3½ pints (1.5–2 liters) of water

For information about exercise and diet after the fat loss plan, turn to pages 150–155.

day 53

This is the last of your 'cardio only' days and, as usual, I'll ask you to run or fast-pace walk. You can swim or cycle, of course, if you prefer. Just make sure the session is 30 minutes long and that you work at 75–80% MHR (7–8/10 RPE).

If you're a regular swimmer, try working with floats. Alternate your sessions so that some incorporate a float for your arms, some use a float for your legs, and some don't use one at all. Training like this will target specific parts of your body. Check the intensity you work at (as above).

eat & drink

breakfast fresh fruit salad with yogurt and seeds *p132* **or** large fruit smoothie *p133*

lunch quinoa salad *p136* **or** Camargue rice salad *p136*

dinner carrot and sweet potato fishcakes with herb salad *p144* **or** steamed fish with salsa and salad *p144*

snacks apple, pear, 1 oz (25 g) sunflower seeds, 1 oz (25 g) raisins **and** (for men) banana, 1 oz (25 g) sunflower seeds, ½ oz (10 g) raisins

drink at least 2½–3½ pints (1.5–2 liters) of water

two-part workout

This is a relatively quick workout for you to perform and at only a moderately high intensity level.

1 cardio

Run or fast-pace walk at a constant pace for 30 minutes. Work at 75–80% MHR (7–8/10 RPE).

2 stretching

End the workout with a lower body stretch (*p23*).

day 54

Come on! One big push for the final day. Give it your best shot. And focus. What is there you could do today to improve your workout? If you can think of anything you've missed before, this is almost your last chance to do it.

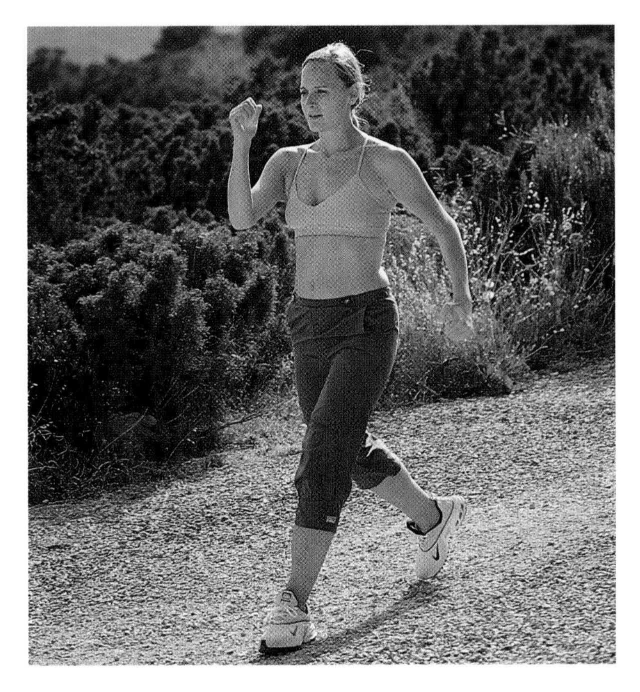

eat&drink

breakfast wheat-free muesli *p132* **or** two slices of whole-wheat toast with nonhydrogenated spread and jam or jelly

lunch asparagus and artichoke salad *p135* **or** green salad *p134*

dinner Thai-style vegetables with polenta *p141* **or** baked zucchini with rice *p140*

snacks apple, pear, and 4 oz (100 g) raspberries or 1 oz (25 g) dried apricots **and** (for men) 1 oz (25 g) mixed sunflower and sesame seeds, 1 oz (25 g) raisins

drink at least 2½–3½ pints (1.5–2 liters) of water

three-part workout

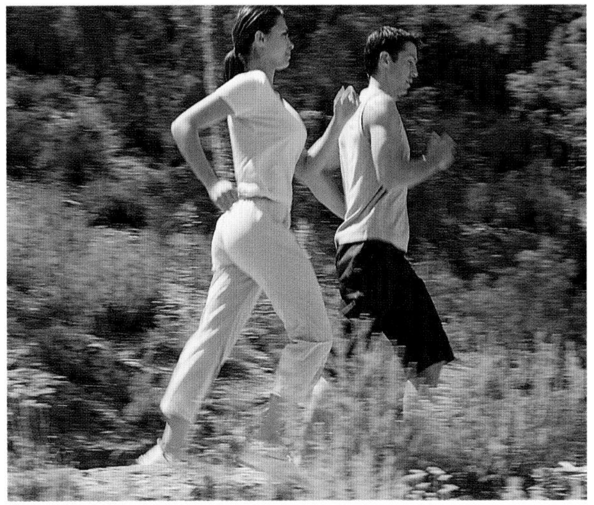

1 cardio

Fast-pace walk for 1 minute, then run for 1 minute. Repeat 11 times, so that you walk and run a total of 12 times each. Run at 90% MHR (9/10 RPE).

During your interval training today, monitor how you feel. How high is your heart rate? How tough are you finding the session? Could you be working any harder? You need to work hard – very hard, in fact – to make the most of this final stage. I'd like you to finish today's workout feeling as though you've given 110%.

2 resistance

Today's resistance is based on PHA, so perform the exercises in order, with 10-second rests between them. After the last one (the oblique bridge), rest for 3 minutes, then repeat the whole sequence twice. As you're doing the exercises, think 'technique, speed, duration, quantity.' Make them perfect and make them hard – what you do today will help you tomorrow.

3 stretching

End today's workout with a total body stretch (*p22*).

day 54 resistance work

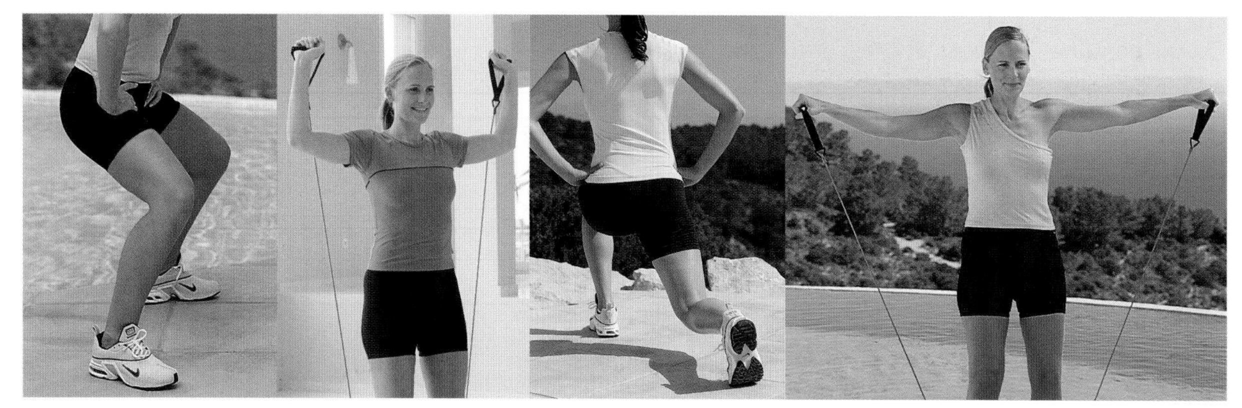

wide squat *p52*
① 25 reps ② 30 reps

shoulder press *p52*
① 15 reps ② 20 reps

walking lunge *p75*
① & ② 20 strides

lateral raise *p21*
① 15 reps ② 20 reps

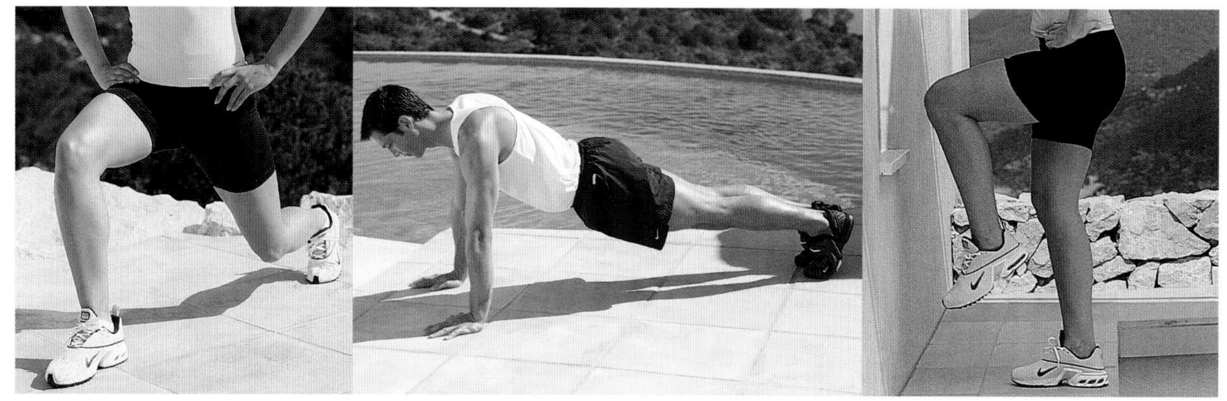

power lunge *p75*
① 15 per leg ② 20 per leg

push-up *p98*
① 12 reps ② 15 reps

knee raise *p92*
① 20 per leg ② 20 per leg

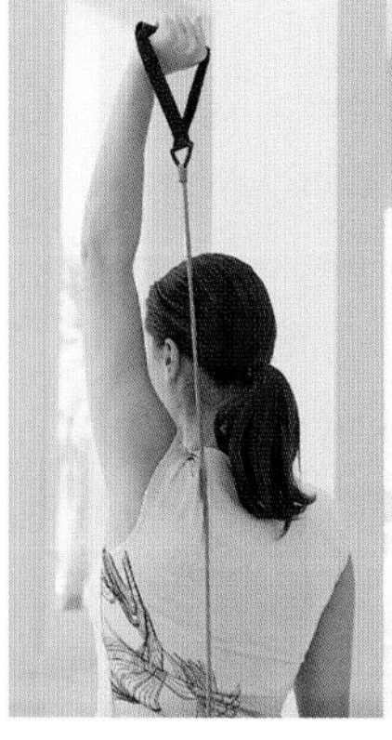

tricep overhead *p103*
① & ② 15 per arm

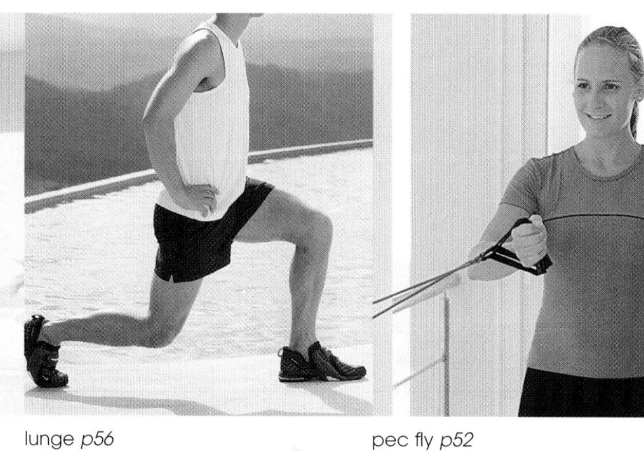

lunge *p56*
① 15 per leg ② 20 per leg

pec fly *p52*
① 12 per arm ② 20 per arm

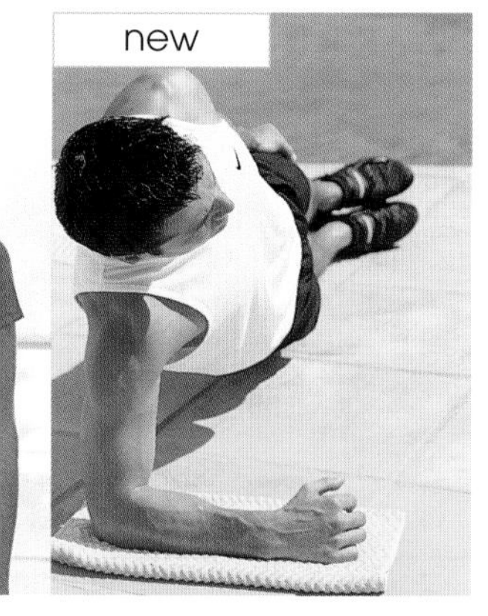

new

oblique bridge *p127*
① & ② 30 secs per side x3

day 54 new exercise

oblique bridge ▷

The most difficult of all exercises for your tummy muscles.

Lie on your side and position your elbow directly under your shoulder for support. Place one foot on top of the other, then raise yourself up, keeping a straight line from your head to your toes. Maintain the position by using your obliques (the muscles at the side of your stomach that run from under your rib cage to your hips). Slowly lower yourself to the start position.

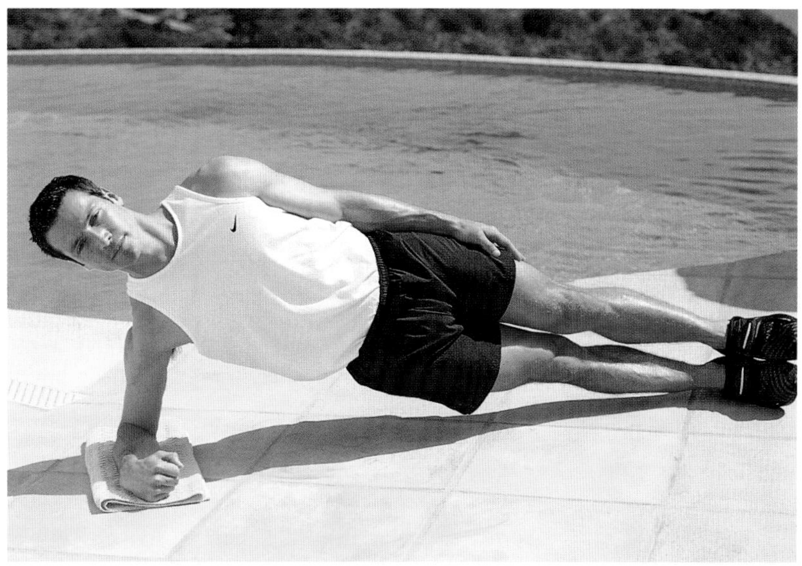

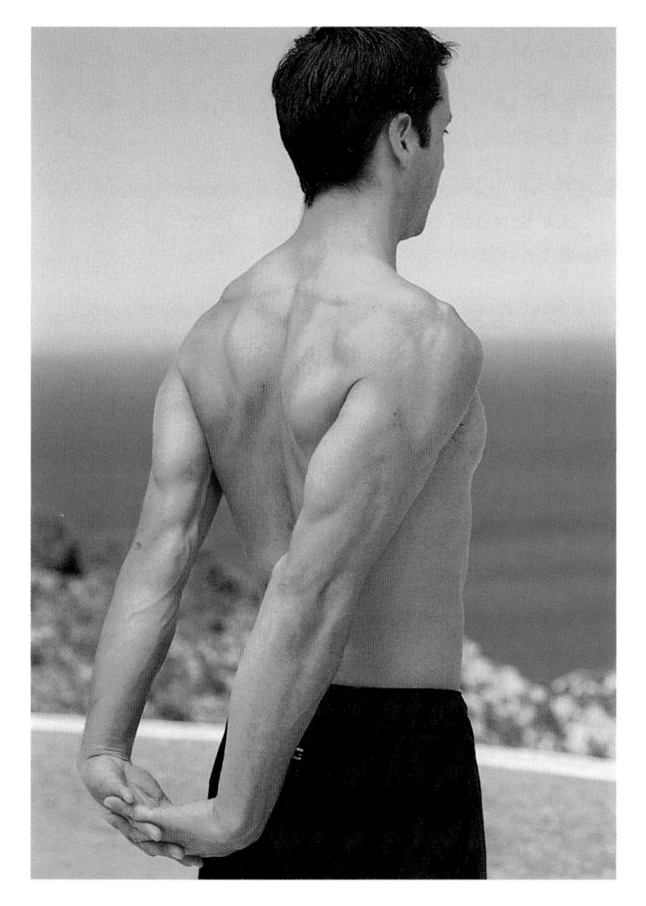

The oblique bridge is difficult, but the **results** are **amazing** – you can create a leaner-looking **waistline** in a very **short** space of time.

◁ After an intense exercise like the oblique bridge, you may want to stretch for a few moments. The chest stretch (*p24*) will help loosen the muscles you used to support your body.

day 55

It's your last rest day of the plan. Devote some time today to thoughts of tomorrow. What are you going to do when you've completed your final workout? Make sure you go out and celebrate. Do something that you've wanted to do for the past eight weeks, but have denied yourself. And enjoy it – in a few days' time you may find yourself setting new goals!

With the help of the plan, you've changed your lifestyle enormously, both in terms of diet and exercise, and in terms of how you think about yourself, too. You may be surprised by the extent to which your body has changed. It's likely you have a new and more positive outlook on life, as well.

Take a little break from exercising after the end of tomorrow. Don't worry too much about your diet. After four days, start planning your next steps. I'll still be with you all the way.

eat & drink

breakfast fresh fruit salad with yogurt and seeds *p132* **or** oatmeal *p132*

lunch broccoli salad *p135* **or** beet and carrot salad *p134*

dinner marinated chicken with steamed vegetables *p149* **or** wheat-free pasta with turkey *p148*

snacks banana, ½ oz (10 g) almonds, 2 oz (50 g) grapes **and** (for men) apple, and 4 oz (100 g) raspberries or 1 oz (25 g) raisins

drink at least 2½–3½ pints (1.5–2 liters) of water

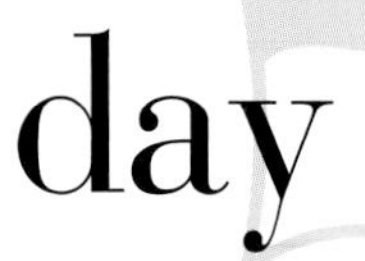

day 56

You may feel as though there's nothing you can do to make a difference on your last day. But you'd be wrong – every little thing you do makes a difference. So stay on the ball. Make your final day a good one. You're now a well-practiced, well-experienced exerciser. You know how to use the information I've given you. Go out and give it your all. Make yourself feel jubilant by completing the plan in its entirety.

eat & drink

breakfast poached egg on two slices of dry whole-wheat toast **or** whole-wheat pancakes *p132*

lunch smoked salmon and dill salad *p138* **or** wild rice salad *p136*

dinner lemon shrimp with three bean salad *p148* **or** Asian stir fry *p141*

snacks apple, pear, 1 oz (25 g) sunflower seeds, 1 oz (25 g) raisins **and** (for men) banana, 1 oz (25 g) sunflower seeds, ½ oz (10 g) raisins

drink at least 2½–3½ pints (1.5–2 liters) of water

three-part workout

Apart from the cardio training, your workout today is a straight repeat of day 54. Before you start the resistance program, run or fast-pace walk at a constant pace for 60 minutes. Work at 70% MHR (7/10 RPE). When you've completed the resistance session, finish the workout with a short standing stretch (*p23*).

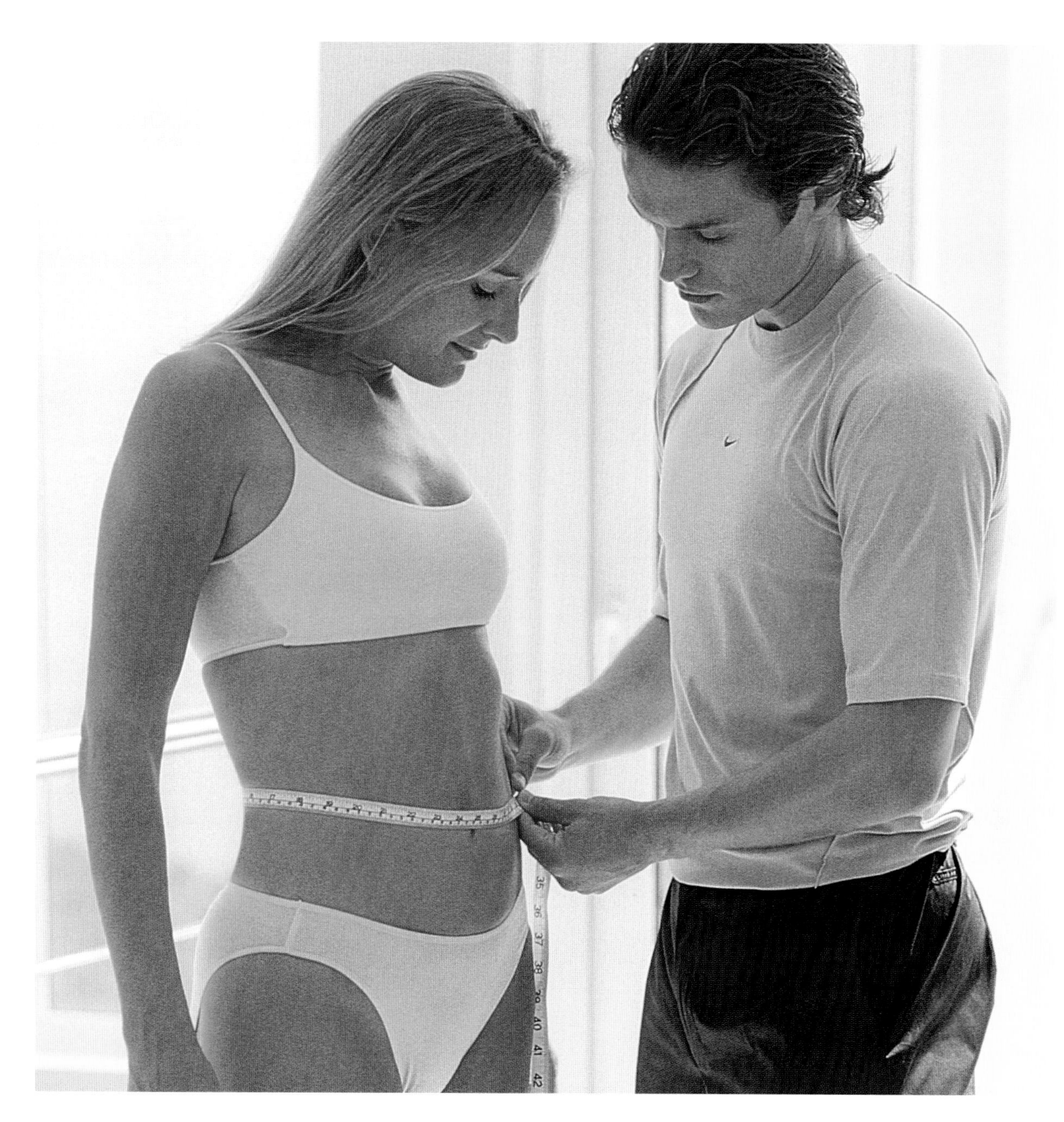

You've done it! You've **completed** the plan. It may be a bit of an anticlimax at first, but now's the time to **set a new goal**. Go for it. Redefine what you thought possible. I wish you **good luck**!

recipes

Whether it's a breakfast, lunch, or dinner dish, each of these calorie-controlled recipes is guaranteed to give you a **delicious** and **healthy** combination of protein, carbs, and fat. What's more, all the meals have been **tried and tested** by **my clients**.

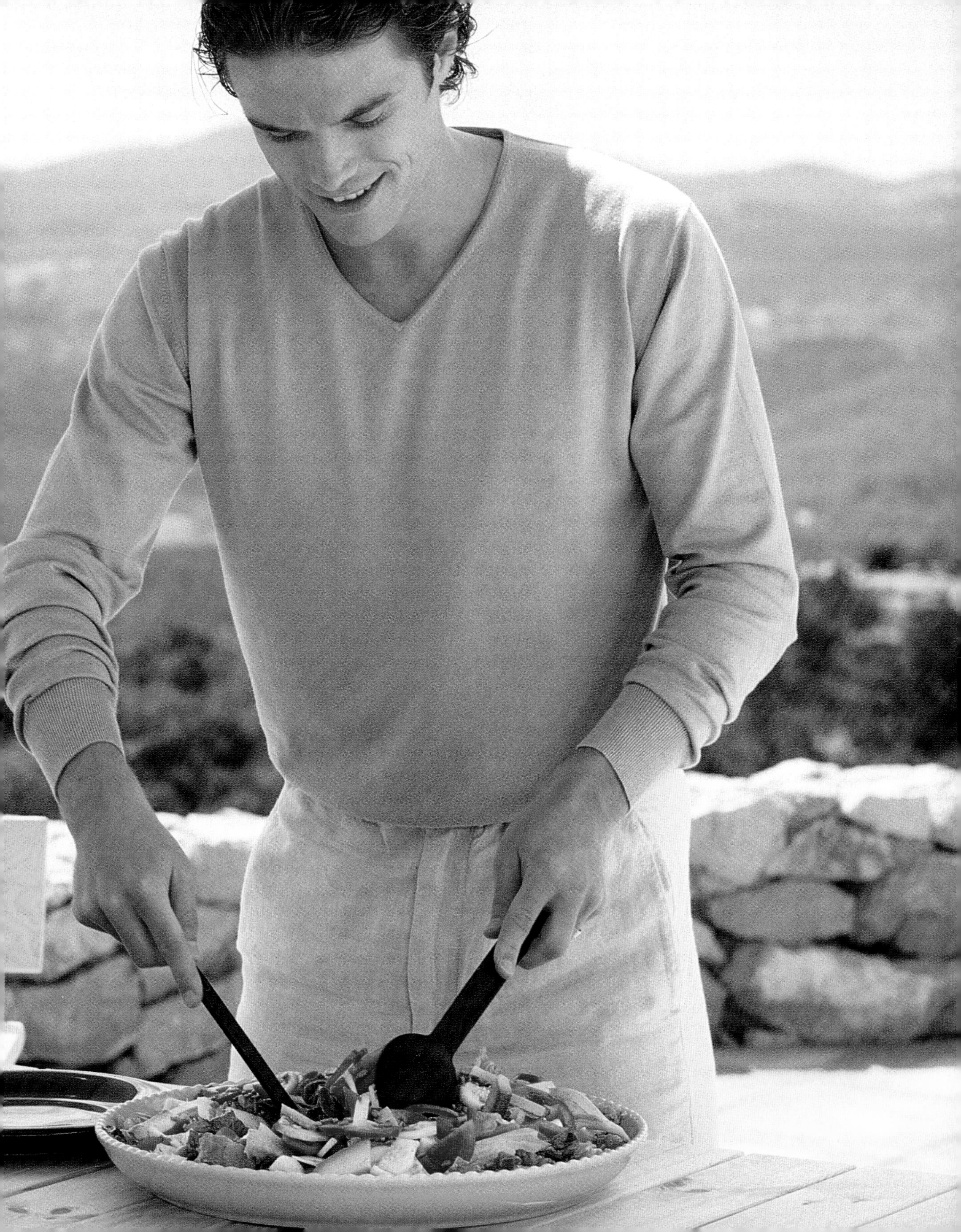

breakfast recipes

wheat-free muesli

① protein ③ carbs ① fat ⓪ saturated fat

3 tbsp rolled oats

2 tbsp puffed rice

1 tbsp puffed millet

1½ tbsp raisins

1 tbsp pumpkin seeds

5 almonds, chopped

2 tsp sesame seeds

Put all the ingredients in a cereal bowl and mix well. Add skim milk or rice milk to taste, and serve immediately.

oatmeal

① protein ③ carbs ⓪ fat ⓪ saturated fat

2 oz/50 g rolled oats

½ pint/300 ml skim milk

for a topping

2 tsp raisins or 2 tsp raspberries or 1 tsp clear honey

1 Pour the milk into a small saucepan and heat until almost boiling. Add the rolled oats and stir for 2–3 minutes until the oatmeal is thick and creamy.

2 Spoon into a cereal bowl and add the topping of your choice.

whole-wheat pancakes

① protein ③ carbs ② fat ① saturated fat

4 oz/100 g whole-wheat flour

7 tbsp skim milk

1 medium-sized egg

1 tsp olive oil

for the filling

2 tbsp plain low-fat yogurt and

1 banana, sliced or

1 apple, sliced or

1 pear, sliced

1 Put the pancake ingredients in a bowl and whisk to a smooth batter.

2 Place a nonstick pan on the stove and allow it to heat up. You'll know when the pan has reached the right temperature because a tiny amount of batter dropped into it will cook through in a few seconds.

3 Pour half the batter into the pan, then tilt the pan from side to side so the batter spreads out into a thick pancake. Cook for 1 minute, then run a spatula around the outside of the pancake to loosen it. Carefully turn the pancake over and cook it on the other side for 1 minute.

4 Slide the pancake onto a serving plate and cover with a clean dish towel to keep warm. Wipe the pan clean, then cook the other half of the batter in the same way.

5 Slide the second pancake onto the plate, and serve with the filling of your choice.

raspberry fool

③ protein ③ carbs ① fat ⓪ saturated fat

6 oz/150 g fresh raspberries

6 oz/150 g plain low-fat yogurt

1 tbsp runny honey

Place the ingredients in a small bowl and mix vigorously with a fork so the raspberries break up and the color spreads through the mixture. Once you have an even consistency, serve immediately.

fresh fruit salad with yogurt and seeds

② protein ③ carbs ① fat ⓪ saturated fat

6 strawberries, hulled

plus any three of the following fruits

1 apple, cut into chunks

1 pear, cut into chunks

1 banana, peeled and cut into chunks

3 fresh apricots, cut in half

2 kiwi fruits, peeled and sliced

6 oz/150 g low-fat plain yogurt

2 tsp sesame seeds

2 tsp sunflower seeds

Place the fruit of your choice in a bowl, then spoon on the yogurt. Sprinkle the seeds over the top, and serve immediately.

vegetable omelet

③ protein ② carbs ① fat ① saturated fat

Making omelets can be a bit of a fine art, I find, and ultimately it comes down to having a really good nonstick pan. This makes them easier to cook and, more importantly, cuts down on the amount of oil you use. This low-cal omelet calls for the whites of the egg only.

3 large egg whites

2 tbsp 1 percent milk

1 tsp olive oil

1 oz/25 g mushrooms, finely chopped

1 oz/25 g red pepper, finely chopped

1 oz/25 g canned corn (drained weight)

1 Place the egg whites in a mixing bowl and add the milk. Whisk well.

2 Place a small nonstick pan on the heat and allow it to get hot. Then coat the inside of the pan with the olive oil.

3 Add the mushrooms and pepper, and cook. When they're soft, and any moisture in the pan has evaporated, add the corn and the egg mix. You should see the outside of the omelet immediately start to set. Gently stir the center so that it doesn't burn.

4 When the underside is cooked, either do as I do and place the pan under a hot broiler to cook the top, or cover it with a lid. Whichever way you choose, it will take only a couple of minutes.

5 Turn the omelet out onto a dinner plate, and season to taste.

large fruit smoothie

① protein ③ carbs ① fat ① saturated fat

Quick and simple to make, this fruit smoothie is packed with vitamins to give your body a boost just when it needs it most – first thing in the morning.

1 banana, cut into chunks

6 strawberries

1½ tbsp blueberries

10 raspberries

⅓ pint/200 ml freshly squeezed orange juice

3 tbsp low-fat plain yogurt

a few small ice cubes

Place the ingredients in your blender, or in a mixing bowl if you're using a hand blender. Blend until smooth. Pour into a glass and serve immediately.

small fruit smoothie

⓪ protein ③ carbs ⓪ fat ⓪ saturated fat

1 banana, cut into chunks

4 strawberries

1 tbsp blueberries

6 raspberries

¼ pint/150 ml freshly squeezed orange juice

a few small ice cubes

Place the ingredients in your blender, or in a mixing bowl if you're using a hand blender. Blend until smooth. Pour into a glass and serve immediately.

smoothie variation

As a delicious alternative to the strawberry, blueberry, and raspberry smoothie, you can substitute pear, kiwi fruit, pineapple, and apple juice.

For the large fruit smoothie, use 1 banana, 1 pear, 3 kiwi fruits, 2 oz/50 g pineapple, and ⅓ pint/200 ml apple juice. Cut the fruit into small chunks. The amount of yogurt remains the same.

For the small fruit smoothie, use 1 banana, 1 pear, 3 kiwi fruits, 1 oz/25 g pineapple (all cut into chunks) and ¼ pint/150 ml apple juice.

nutrition key

The ideal fat loss breakfast is high in slow-release complex carbs (carbohydrates). There's a small amount of protein, too, to pep up your brain in the morning.

⓪ negligible or none

① low

② medium

③ high

lunch recipes

green salad

① protein ② carbs ① fat ⓪ saturated fat

2 oz/50 g green beans, trimmed

2 oz/50 g peas (shelled weight)

3 oz/75 g broccoli, cut into florets

3 oz/75 g zucchini, thickly sliced

2 oz/50 g snow peas, trimmed

3 oz/75 g mixed salad leaves and herbs

2 oz/50 g canned cannellini beans (drained weight)

for the dressing

1 tbsp fat-free yogurt

2 tsp finely chopped fresh basil

½ tsp wholegrain mustard

1 Boil or steam the vegetables (first five ingredients) until tender.

2 Make the dressing by putting the ingredients in a cup or small bowl and whisking together until blended.

3 Arrange the salad leaves and herbs on a dinner plate.

4 When the vegetables are cooked, drain well, then mix together in a bowl. Add the drained cannellini beans and mix again.

5 Drizzle over the dressing, then toss until all the ingredients are evenly coated with it.

6 Pile the vegetables onto the salad leaves, season to taste, and serve immediately.

beet and carrot salad

① protein ③ carbs ① fat ⓪ saturated fat

6 oz/150 g cooked beets, cubed

4 oz/100 g raw carrot, grated

4 oz/100 g canned cranberry beans or cannellini beans (drained weight)

3 oz/75 g celery, finely sliced

2 oz/50 g quinoa, cooked according to the packet instructions

for the dressing

2 tsp olive oil

1 tsp balsamic vinegar

a few fresh basil leaves, torn into strips

1 Place all the salad ingredients in a serving bowl and mix together well.

2 Make the dressing by whisking the oil and vinegar together in a small bowl and then adding the basil.

3 Pour the dressing over the salad and toss so that all the ingredients are evenly coated. Season to taste and serve.

Greek salad

① protein ③ carbs ② fat ① saturated fat

50 g/2 oz feta cheese, cubed

5 butterhead lettuce leaves, cleaned and shredded into small pieces

5 baby plum tomatoes, cut lengthwise into quarters

50 g/2 oz green and/or yellow bell pepper, sliced

6 green olives, pitted and sliced

½ small red onion, peeled and thinly sliced

25 g/1 oz cucumber, diced

50 g/2 oz canned red kidney beans (drained weight)

for the dressing

2 tsp olive oil

2 tsp freshly squeezed lemon juice

1 Place the salad ingredients in a serving bowl and mix together well.

2 Make the dressing by whisking the olive oil and lemon juice together.

3 Drizzle the dressing over the salad and toss so that all the ingredients are evenly coated. Season to taste and serve immediately.

broccoli salad

① protein ③ carbs ② fat ⓪ saturated fat

50 g/2 oz broccoli, cut into florets

50 g/2 oz cauliflower, cut into florets

50 g/2 oz green beans, trimmed

25 g/1 oz baby carrots, scrubbed and trimmed

25 g/1 oz baby corn cobs, trimmed

25 g/1 oz sugar snap peas, trimmed

40 g/1½ oz baby butternut squash or zucchini, cut into chunks

60g /2½ oz canned green lentils (drained weight)

2 tsp sesame seeds

for the dressing

2 tsp sesame oil

1 tsp olive oil

2 tsp white wine vinegar

1 Cook the broccoli and cauliflower florets in a pan of boiling water until cooked but still slightly crunchy. Remove with a slotted spoon and plunge immediately into a bowl of ice-cold water to stop the cooking.

2 Repeat the process, using the same pan of water to cook the beans, carrots, and baby corn together. Transfer them to the ice water and then cook the peas and squash or zucchini in the same way.

3 Make the dressing by putting the ingredients in a cup or bowl and whisking them together.

4 Drain the cooked vegetables well, then pat dry with a paper towel.

5 Transfer the vegetables to a bowl, add the lentils, sesame seeds, and dressing. Toss to coat the ingredients evenly, then season to taste. Serve immediately.

asparagus and artichoke salad

① protein ③ carbs ① fat ⓪ saturated fat

The dressing for this salad has a gutsy flavor that comes from roasting the tomatoes yourself. You may feel it's not worth switching your oven on just for them – but they're fine cooked and prepared the day before if that's more convenient. If you're really pressed for time, however, you can substitute fresh tomato juice – the flavor will still be good, though not quite so good.

6 asparagus spears

5 artichoke hearts canned in water, drained and cut into quarters

2 oz/50 g mushrooms, finely sliced

2 oz/50 g apple, finely diced

2 oz/50 g celery, thinly sliced

3 oz/75 g canned lima beans (drained weight)

50 g/2 oz celery root or carrot, peeled and grated

for the dressing

2 plum tomatoes (or 2 tbsp tomato juice)

1 tbsp carrot juice

1 tsp olive oil

½ tsp wholegrain mustard

1 Preheat the oven to 450° F/230° C. Meanwhile, trim the asparagus spears, then steam or boil for 7–10 minutes until tender.

2 Make the dressing by placing the tomatoes in a baking pan and roasting in the preheated oven for about 5–10 minutes. Once they're starting to char on the outside and look soft, take them out of the oven and use the back of a wooden spoon to push them through a sieve placed over a small bowl so you catch all the delicious juices – these are the base for your dressing.

3 If you're using fresh tomato juice, spoon it into a bowl.

4 Add the other dressing ingredients to your tomato juice, then whisk well.

5 Place all the salad ingredients except the asparagus in a serving bowl and drizzle with dressing. Mix to coat the ingredients evenly.

6 Place the cooked asparagus spears on top, season to taste, and serve immediately.

nutrition key

The ideal lunch for fat loss is high in carbs, to fuel you through the afternoon. There's some protein, too. Don't be alarmed by lunches that I've marked as 'high' in fat, by the way. This is the total fat content of the dish and includes all the polyunsaturated and unsaturated fats that speed up our metabolisms and help our bodies produce energy. It's the saturated fat score that matters. These are the fats that slow down our bodies. In my recipes, the saturated fat content is always low or zero.

⓪ negligible or none

① low

② medium

③ high

wild rice salad

① protein ③ carbs ② fat ⓪ saturated fat

The dressing for this salad is great for making in larger quantities. Store it in an airtight container in the fridge – it'll keep for a week or so – and then use it on any leaf salad.

2 oz/50 g wild rice, cooked according to the packet instructions

1 tbsp sesame seeds

2 oz/50 g canned red kidney beans (drained weight)

2 oz/50 g ripe avocado, peeled and cubed

2 oz/50 g bean sprouts, cut in half

1 oz/25 g walnuts, chopped finely

for the dressing

5 raspberries

1 tsp raspberry vinegar

1 tsp olive oil

½ tsp soy sauce

1 Place the salad ingredients in a serving bowl.

2 Make the dressing by placing the raspberries and the vinegar in a small bowl. Crush the raspberries with a fork, and then whisk in the oil and soy sauce. (Alternatively, you can use a mortar and pestle to do this.)

3 Drizzle the dressing over the salad. Toss to coat the ingredients evenly, season to taste, and serve.

Camargue rice salad

① protein ③ carbs ① fat ⓪ saturated fat

I find this salad is even better if you leave it for a little while after you've made it – the flavors have more time to work together. For that very reason, I often make it first thing in the morning, or even the night before, and then store it in an airtight container in the fridge. Make sure you take it out of the fridge, though, about 30 minutes before you plan to eat it so it has time to reach room temperature.

2 oz/50 g red Camargue rice or other wholegrain rice, cooked according to packet instructions

1½ oz/35 g carrot, scrubbed and grated

1½ oz/35 g zucchini, grated

1 scallion, finely chopped

2 oz/50 g red bell pepper, finely chopped

2 oz/50 g canned green lentils (drained weight)

for the dressing

1 tsp olive oil

1 tsp balsamic vinegar

½ tsp sherry vinegar

½ tsp crushed garlic

1 Place all the salad ingredients in a serving bowl and mix together well.

2 Make the dressing by putting the ingredients in a cup or bowl and whisking them together well.

3 Drizzle the dressing over the salad. Toss to coat the ingredients well, season to taste, and serve.

quinoa salad

① protein ③ carbs ① fat ⓪ saturated fat

This dish uses the South American grain quinoa (pronounced *keen-wah*). Highly nutritious, quick to cook, and very easy for the body to digest, quinoa is available in most good supermarkets, although you may need to search for it a bit.

4 oz/100 g quinoa, cooked according to the packet instructions

3 oz/75 g ripe mango, peeled and cubed

2 oz/50 g canned sweetcorn (drained weight)

1 oz/25 g canned chick peas (drained weight)

25 g/1 oz red bell pepper, finely chopped

2 tsp finely chopped fresh mint

for the dressing

2 tbsp carrot juice

2 tsp olive oil

1 tsp wholegrain mustard

1 tsp freshly squeezed lime juice

1 Put all the salad ingredients in a serving bowl and mix together well.

2 Make the dressing by putting all the ingredients in a cup or bowl and whisking until smooth.

3 Drizzle the dressing over the salad. Mix to coat the ingredients evenly, season to taste, and serve.

shrimp and linguine salad

(2) protein (3) carbs (2) fat (0) saturated fat

3 oz/75 g cooked shrimp, shelled

1½ oz/35 g fresh or dried linguine

2 oz/50 g leek, cleaned and sliced

1 tbsp white wine

for the dressing

2 tsp freshly squeezed lemon juice

2 tsp olive oil

2 tsp very finely chopped fresh rosemary or ½ tsp finely chopped dried rosemary

1 Make the dressing by mixing the lemon juice, olive oil, and rosemary in a small bowl.

2 With a knife, make a slit along the back of each shrimp. This gives them a better texture for eating and makes them look more attractive. Rinse them clean in running water, then pat dry with a paper towel.

3 Heat a non stick skillet and put the leeks in to fry. If they start to stick, add a little water.

4 Meanwhile, put the linguine on to cook according to the instructions on the packet.

5 When the leeks are cooked and any liquid has evaporated, add the white wine. Allow to bubble, then add the shrimp and heat through until they open out.

6 Drain the cooked linguine well, then transfer to a serving bowl and drizzle with the dressing.

7 Add the shrimp, leeks, and cooking liquor to the linguine, then mix well and season to taste.

salade niçoise

(3) protein (2) carbs (2) fat (0) saturated fat

Traditionally, a salade niçoise is built up gradually, with one layer of ingredients added at a time. We need to add as much flavor to the dish as possible, however, since we are using a lot less dressing. Tossing most of the ingredients well first in a bowl will really help mix up the flavors.

4 oz/100 g fresh tuna, grilled, or tuna canned in spring water, drained

2 oz/50 g small new potatoes, scrubbed

2 oz/50 g green beans, trimmed

5 butterhead lettuce leaves, cleaned

3 plum tomatoes

1 tbsp capers in brine, drained

6 black olives, pitted

4 anchovy filets in olive oil, drained

½ small red onion, peeled and roughly chopped

5 basil leaves

for the dressing

1 tbsp olive oil

2 tsp balsamic vinegar

1 Steam or boil the potatoes and beans until tender.

2 Meanwhile, arrange the lettuce leaves in a fan shape in the center of a dinner plate.

3 Make the dressing by mixing the oil and vinegar together in a cup or bowl and then set aside.

4 Slice the tomatoes lengthwise into quarters and place them in a mixing bowl. Finely chop the capers, olives, and anchovies and add them to the bowl.

5 Halve the cooked potatoes (or leave whole if really small) and add to the bowl along with the beans and onion. Tear the basil leaves into small pieces and add them, too.

6 Sprinkle the dressing over the ingredients and toss to coat evenly. Allow the salad to stand for a few minutes so the flavors of the basil, anchovy, and capers infuse through the entire mix.

7 Spoon the salad and any juices onto the lettuce and season to taste. Last of all, break the tuna into chunks and arrange them on the top.

nutrition key

(0) negligible or none

(1) low

(2) medium

(3) high

smoked salmon and dill salad

③ protein ② carbs ② fat ⓪ saturated fat

4 oz/100 g smoked salmon, cut into long, thin strips

6 oz/150 g small new potatoes, scrubbed

2 oz/50 g cucumber, finely diced

2 oz/50 g arugula

2 oz/50 g herb salad or mix of aromatic salad leaves

2 tsp freshly squeezed lemon juice

for the dressing

1 tbsp finely chopped fresh dill

2 tbsp plain fat-free yogurt

2 tsp freshly squeezed lemon juice

1 Steam or boil the potatoes until tender.

2 Make the dressing by putting the ingredients in a small bowl and mixing with a spoon so the flavors blend. Add the salmon and cucumber and mix well.

3 Arrange the arugula and salad around the outside of a dinner plate.

4 Slice the cooked potatoes (or leave whole if small) and place in the middle of the salad, then drizzle the lemon juice over the potatoes and salad.

5 Arrange the salmon and cucumber mixture on top of the potatoes. Season with black pepper, but go lightly on the salt because smoked salmon is already salty.

tuna sandwich

③ protein ① carbs ② fat ⓪ saturated fat

4 oz/100 g tuna canned in water or brine (drained weight)

2 slices whole-wheat bread

½ small red onion, peeled and finely chopped

1 tomato, finely chopped

3 drops hot pepper sauce such as Tabasco

1 tbsp low-fat cottage cheese

1 Place the tuna, onion, tomato, and hot pepper sauce in a mixing bowl and mix together well.

2 To assemble your sandwich, spread the cottage cheese on one slice of bread. Spread the tuna mixture evenly over it, and then top with the other slice of bread. Cut in half to serve.

cottage cheese, cranberry, and arugula sandwich

② protein ② carbs ② fat ① saturated fat

6 oz/150 g low-fat cottage cheese

4 tbsp cranberry sauce

2 oz/50 g arugula

cholesterol-free mayonnaise, thinly spread

4 slices whole-wheat bread

1 Spread a scraping of cholesterol-free mayonnaise on each of the four slices of bread.

2 Spread the cottage cheese on two of the pieces and cranberry sauce on the others.

3 Divide the arugula between the pieces of bread spread with cottage cheese, then place the pieces spread with cranberry sauce on top.

4 Cut each sandwich in half, and enjoy!

smoked salmon sandwich

② protein ② carbs ③ fat ① saturated fat

4 oz/100 g smoked salmon

2 slices whole-wheat bread

4 oz/100 g low-fat cottage cheese

2 oz/50 g arugula

whole grain mustard to taste

1 To assemble your sandwich, spread the cottage cheese over one slice of bread. Arrange the arugula on top of it, and then place the smoked salmon on top of that.

2 Dab with a small amount of mustard here and there, then top with the other slice of bread. Cut in half to serve.

broiled vegetable pitas

② protein ② carbs ③ fat ① saturated fat

These sandwiches are equally good hot or cold. You can even make them the night before and store them in the refrigerator until about 30 minutes before you're ready to eat them. You need to work slightly ahead anyway – an essential part of this recipe is marinating the vegetables for about half an hour.

½ zucchini, cut into long, thin slices

4 small, thin asparagus spears

1 small red bell pepper, cut into long, thin slices

1 whole-wheat pita bread

2 oz/50 g low-fat cream cheese

for the marinade

1 tbsp balsamic vinegar

1 tsp finely chopped fresh thyme or ½ tsp dried thyme

1 tsp Dijon mustard

1 tbsp olive oil

4 tbsp vegetable stock (made from vegetable bouillon powder or a vegetable stock cube)

2 tsp finely chopped fresh basil

1 Make the marinade by whisking the ingredients together in a bowl.

2 Place the prepared raw vegetables in a large, flat-bottomed dish and pour over the marinade. Stir every few minutes so they marinate evenly. Leave them for about 20–30 minutes.

3 Preheat the broiler. Remove the vegetables from the marinade with a slotted spoon and place them on a broiler pan.

4 Broil the vegetables on a medium to high heat for about 2–3 minutes on each side, or until they're just starting to brown.

5 When the vegetables are nearly cooked, toast the pita until golden brown. Allow it to cool slightly.

6 Slice the toasted pita open down one edge to make a pocket. Then spread the cream cheese evenly on the inside surfaces.

7 To assemble your sandwich, build up layers of cooked vegetables inside the pita, starting with the red pepper, and finishing with the asparagus spears. Press gently together, then cut in half to serve.

nutrition key

⓪ negligible or none

① low

② medium

③ high

dinner recipes

baked zucchini with rice

① protein ③ carbs ① fat ⓪ saturated fat

1 large zucchini

4 oz/100 g wholegrain rice

3 small mushrooms, finely sliced

1 plum tomato, chopped

6 cashew nuts, finely chopped

1 tsp finely chopped fresh rosemary or ½ tsp finely chopped dried rosemary

1 tsp finely chopped fresh basil

2 tsp olive oil

1 tsp balsamic vinegar

1 tsp freshly squeezed lemon juice

1 Preheat the oven to 350° F/180° C. Meanwhile, top and tail the zucchini and halve lengthwise. Use a teaspoon to scoop out most of the insides to make two shells. Chop half the removed flesh; discard the rest.

2 Put the chopped zucchini in a mixing bowl. Add the mushrooms, tomato, cashew nuts, rosemary, basil, olive oil, balsamic vinegar, and lemon juice. Mix, then spoon into the shells.

3 Put the rice on to cook according to the packet instructions.

4 Fifteen minutes before the rice is due to be ready, place the zucchini in the preheated oven and bake for 15 minutes, or until the zucchini is just beginning to soften.

5 When the rice is cooked, drain then arrange on a plate. Place the zucchini on top, season and serve.

sweet potato gnocchi with tomato and shrimp sauce

③ protein ③ carbs ① fat ⓪ saturated fat

2 small to medium sweet potatoes

2 oz/50 g whole-wheat flour (plus a little extra for shaping)

1½ tsp ground nutmeg

for the sauce

9 oz/225 g canned chopped tomatoes and their juice

3 oz/75 g cooked shrimp

1 tsp olive oil

1 tsp chopped garlic

1½ oz/35 g onion, peeled and finely chopped

1½ oz/35 g mushrooms, finely chopped

1 tbsp red wine (optional)

1 tsp finely chopped fresh oregano or ½ tsp dried oregano

2 tsp finely chopped fresh basil

1 Preheat the oven to 350° F/180° C.

2 Roast the sweet potatoes in the preheated oven for about 35 minutes, or until the flesh is soft when pierced with a skewer. Allow to cool slightly, then remove the skin.

3 Put the sweet potato flesh in a mixing bowl – you should have about 7 oz/175 g of it. Add the flour and mash thoroughly so you have a smooth mixture. Add the nutmeg and mix again. Season lightly.

4 Sprinkle a little flour on a clean work surface. Lightly coat your hands with it. Take some gnocchi mixture – an amount about the size of a brazil nut – and gently roll it in your hands and on the floured surface until you have a ball; flatten slightly with a fork. Place it on one side. Repeat the process until you've used up all the mixture. Then put the gnocchi in the fridge for half an hour or so while you prepare the sauce.

5 Make the sauce by heating the olive oil in a non stick skillet. Add the garlic and onion and cook until soft. Add the mushrooms, and a little water if the pan is getting dry. When the mushrooms are starting to soften, add the red wine (or 1 tbsp water). Let the mixture bubble for a few moments before adding the oregano.

6 Now add the tomatoes and juice. Stir well so the tomatoes disintegrate in the sauce. Finally, add the shrimp and stir well. Turn the heat down and allow to simmer for 15–20 minutes, stirring occasionally. The sauce should reduce to a thick consistency. Add the basil.

7 Just before the sauce is due to be ready, place the gnocchi one by one in a large pan of boiling water and cook for about 3 minutes. They'll rise to the surface when they're cooked.

8 With a slotted spoon, transfer the gnocchi to a dinner plate. Top with the sauce. Season to taste, and serve immediately.

Asian stir fry

② protein ② carbs ① fat ⓪ saturated fat

3 oz/75 g skinless chicken breast or tofu, cut into cubes

6 oz/150 g whole-wheat noodles, cooked according to the packet instructions

1 tsp sesame oil

1 tsp finely minced garlic

2 tsp peeled and finely minced fresh root ginger

2 tsp soy sauce

½ tsp chili paste

2 tsp freshly squeezed lime juice

2 oz/50 g carrot, cut into thin sticks

1½ oz/35 g leek, cleaned and sliced

2 oz/50 g mushrooms, sliced

2 oz/50 g snow peas, halved

1½ oz/35 g bean sprouts

2 oz/50 g green cabbage, shredded

1 Heat a wok or frying pan, add the sesame oil, and put the garlic and ginger in to fry. Turn the heat down so they don't burn. After a minute, add the chicken or tofu and stir so they don't stick (if they do, add 1–2 tbsp hot water). Add the soy sauce and chili paste, stirring constantly.

2 Once the chicken or tofu has browned slightly, add the lime juice, carrot, and leek. Cook, stirring all the time, for 2 minutes, then add the mushrooms and 2 tbsp hot water.

3 When the mushrooms have softened, add the snow peas. Continue to stir. After a minute, add the bean sprouts. Cook, stirring, for another minute before adding the cabbage. Allow the ingredients to cook for 2 minutes. Season to taste, and serve with the cooked noodles.

Thai-style vegetables with polenta

⓪ protein ③ carbs ① fat ⓪ saturated fat

3 oz/75 g button mushrooms

4 oz/100 g red and/or green bell pepper, deseeded and cut into large chunks

3 oz/75 g zucchini, cut into large chunks

4 baby corn cobs

2 oz/50 g polenta

12 fl oz/350 ml skim milk

2 tsp finely chopped fresh cilantro

for the marinade

2 tsp peeled and finely minced fresh root ginger

2 tsp finely chopped fresh cilantro

½ tsp deseeded and finely chopped medium-hot red chili

2 tsp freshly squeezed lime juice

2 tbsp soy sauce

4 tbsp water

1 tbsp sesame oil

1 Make the marinade by whisking the ingredients together in a bowl.

2 Place the mushrooms, pepper, zucchini, and baby corn in a flat-bottomed dish and pour the marinade over. Stir well, then leave to stand for 15–30 minutes. Move the vegetables around in the marinade every few minutes so they take on maximum flavor.

3 Preheat the broiler to hot. Remove the vegetables from the marinade and thread onto two skewers. Broil for about 8 minutes, turning the kabobs from time to time so they cook on all sides.

4 Meanwhile, pour the milk into a saucepan and heat until warm but not boiling. Stirring constantly, sprinkle in the polenta and cilantro and cook for a couple of minutes until the polenta is the consistency of mashed potato. Remove immediately from the heat.

5 Spoon the polenta onto a dinner plate. Arrange the vegetable kabobs alongside. Season to taste and serve immediately.

nutrition key

The ideal fat loss dinner has more protein than lunch, and is lighter to digest. As with the lunch dishes, don't be alarmed by recipes that I've marked as 'high' in fat. This is the total fat content of the dish and includes all the polyunsaturated and unsaturated fats that speed up our metabolisms and help our bodies produce energy. It's the saturated fat score that matters. These are the fats that slow down our bodies. In my recipes, the saturated fat content is low or zero.

⓪ negligible or none
① low
② medium
③ high

stuffed bell pepper

① protein ② carbs ① fat ⓪ saturated fat

1 large red bell pepper

2 oz/50 g quinoa

2 oz/50 g mushrooms, finely chopped

3 tsp finely chopped fresh thyme or 1 tsp dried thyme

2 tsp freshly squeezed lemon juice

3 oz/75 g tomato, finely chopped

2 oz/50 g eggplant, cut into cubes

1 tsp olive oil

2 tsp freshly grated Parmesan cheese

1 Preheat the oven to 450° F/230° C.

2 Cook the quinoa according to the packet instructions.

3 Meanwhile, halve the pepper lengthwise and remove the seeds. Leave the stalk as decoration.

4 Once the quinoa is cooked, drain it and put it in a bowl with all the other ingredients except the Parmesan. Mix together well, then spoon the mixture into the halved peppers.

5 Place the stuffed peppers on a baking dish, sprinkle with Parmesan cheese, and bake in the preheated oven for 25 minutes.

6 Place the stuffed peppers on a dinner plate. Season to taste and serve.

mushroom risotto

① protein ③ carbs ② fat ① saturated fat

½ oz/15 g dried porcini mushrooms

2 oz/50 g fresh mushrooms, finely chopped

4 oz/100 g risotto rice

1 tsp olive oil

½ red onion, finely diced

½ garlic clove, finely minced

½ pint/300 ml vegetable stock (made from bouillon powder or a cube)

2 tsp finely chopped fresh thyme or 1 tsp dried thyme

2 tbsp red wine (optional)

2 tsp freshly grated Parmesan

2 tsp finely chopped fresh parsley

1 Soak the porcini in a small bowl of warm water for 30 minutes, then drain (reserving the liquid) and chop small.

2 Heat the oil in a saucepan and fry the onion and garlic for 5 minutes. In a separate saucepan, heat the stock.

3 Add the porcini and thyme to the onions. If they start to stick, add a little hot water. Two minutes later, add the rice, then stir for 2–3 minutes. Add the wine and reserved liquid.

4 Stirring constantly, add a ladleful of hot stock to the pan. Add another as soon as the previous one has been absorbed, and so on until the stock is used. Add the mushrooms and stir.

5 Cook until the mushrooms are tender and the rice is *al dente* (check the packet instructions for timings). The risotto should be moist.

6 Take the risotto from the heat, and stir in the Parmesan and parsley. Transfer to a dinner plate, season to taste, and serve.

vegetable and tofu kabobs

② protein ③ carbs ③ fat ① saturated fat

6 oz/150 g tofu or smoked tofu, cut into 1 in/2.5 cm cubes

50 g/2 oz red and/or yellow bell pepper, deseeded and cut into squares

2 oz/50 g eggplant, cut into cubes

6 cherry tomatoes

2 oz/50 g zucchini, cut into chunks

3 oz/75 g wholegrain rice, cooked according to the packet instructions

for the marinade

1 tbsp balsamic vinegar

1 tsp chopped fresh thyme or ½ tsp dried thyme

1 tbsp Dijon mustard

2 tsp olive oil

½ pint/300 ml vegetable stock (made from bouillon powder or a cube)

1 Make the marinade by placing all the ingredients in a bowl and whisking them together well.

2 Place the prepared vegetables and tofu in a flat-bottomed dish and pour the marinade over. Leave to marinate for about an hour, stirring the ingredients occasionally.

3 Preheat the broiler to hot. Meanwhile, remove the vegetables and tofu from the marinade and thread on to two kabob skewers.

4 Place the kabobs under the preheated broiler and cook for about 12 minutes, turning occasionally.

5 Arrange the rice on a dinner plate and place the kabobs on top. Season to taste and serve immediately.

salmon and vegetable kabobs

② protein ③ carbs ① fat ⓪ saturated fat

4 oz/100 g fresh salmon steak, skinned and cut into cubes

1 oz/25 g each green and red bell pepper, deseeded and cut into squares

4 large mushrooms

2 baby corns, cut in half crosswise

2 oz/50 g wholegrain rice, cooked according to the packet instructions

for the marinade

1 tbsp honey

½ pint/300 ml warm water

¼ pint/125 ml dry white wine

2 tbsp freshly squeezed lemon juice

2 tsp olive oil

2 tbsp chopped fresh rosemary or 1 tbsp chopped dried rosemary

1 Make the marinade by dissolving the honey in the warm water in a bowl. Add the other ingredients and stir well. Allow to cool.

2 Add the salmon and vegetables to the cooled marinade and stir well. Cover with plastic wrap, place in the fridge, and leave for at least 2 hours and up to 24 hours. Stir occasionally.

3 Preheat the broiler to hot. Remove the salmon and vegetables from the marinade and thread onto two kabob skewers. Place the kabobs under the broiler and cook for 3–5 minutes on each side, or until the salmon and vegetables are cooked.

4 Arrange the cooked rice on a dinner plate and place the kabobs on top. Season to taste and serve.

chicken and vegetable kabobs

② protein ③ carbs ③ fat ① saturated fat

6 oz/150 g skinless, boneless chicken breast, cut into 1 in/2.5 cm cubes

2 oz/50 g red or yellow bell pepper, deseeded and cut into squares

2 oz/50 g eggplant, cut into cubes

6 cherry tomatoes

2 oz/50 g zucchini, cut into chunks

3 oz/75 g wholegrain rice, cooked according to packet instructions

for the marinade

1 tbsp balsamic vinegar

1 tsp chopped fresh thyme or ½ tsp dried thyme

1 tbsp Dijon mustard

2 tsp olive oil

½ pint/300 ml cold chicken stock (fresh or made from a bouillon cube)

1 Make the marinade by placing all the ingredients in a bowl and whisking them together well.

2 Place the prepared vegetables and chicken in a flat-bottomed dish and pour the marinade over. Leave to marinate for about an hour, stirring the ingredients occasionally.

3 Preheat the broiler to hot. Meanwhile, remove the vegetables and chicken from the marinade and thread onto two kabob skewers.

4 Place the kabobs under the preheated broiler and cook for about 12 minutes, turning to cook evenly.

5 Arrange the cooked rice on a dinner plate and place the kabobs on top. Season to taste and serve immediately.

broiled or steamed fish with quinoa

② protein ③ carbs ② fat ⓪ saturated fat

You can use your favorite kind of fish for this dish (I've given you a list of possible options). Broil it or steam it, as you wish.

8 oz/200 g salmon, snapper, grouper, mahi mahi, or bass (boned weight)

4 oz/100 g quinoa

3 oz/75 g red and/or yellow bell pepper, deseeded and finely diced

3 oz/75 g canned corn (drained weight)

for the dressing

½ tsp Chinese five spice powder

2 tsp freshly squeezed lemon juice

1 tbsp finely chopped fresh cilantro

1 Prepare the quinoa according to the packet instructions, then transfer to a mixing bowl. While it's still warm, mix in the pepper and sweetcorn.

2 Meanwhile, broil or steam the fish of your choice until cooked.

3 Make the dressing by mixing the ingredients together in a small bowl. Drizzle over the quinoa salad.

4 Put the salad on a plate, arrange the fish on top, and season to taste.

nutrition key

⓪ negligible or none

① low

② medium

③ high

steamed fish with salsa and salad

③ protein ① carbs ② fat ⓪ saturated fat

6 oz/150 g firm white fish, such as halibut, snapper, grouper, mahi mahi, or sea bass

3 asparagus spears, trimmed

2 oz/50 g carrot, peeled and sliced

4 oz/100 g canned green lentils (drained weight)

2 large scallions, finely chopped

1 oz/25 g cucumber, finely diced

a few fresh basil leaves

1 tsp olive oil

for the salsa

3 oz/75 g tomato, skinned and finely chopped

1 oz/25 g onion, peeled and finely chopped

1 tsp finely chopped fresh oregano or ½ tsp dried oregano

½ tsp ground cumin

2 tsp freshly squeezed lemon juice

1 tsp freshly squeezed lime juice

4 drops hot sauce like Tabasco

½ tsp chopped garlic

1 Make the salsa by placing the ingredients in a bowl and stirring well.

2 Put the fish of your choice on to steam. Meanwhile, boil or steam the asparagus and carrot.

3 Put the carrot, lentils, scallions, and cucumber in a bowl and mix well. Tear the basil into fine shreds, mix with the olive oil, then drizzle over the salad and toss well.

4 Arrange the salad, asparagus, and fish on a dinner plate, then spoon on the salsa and serve.

carrot and sweet potato fishcakes with herb salad

② protein ② carbs ① fat ⓪ saturated fat

You can use any firm white fish for these fishcakes – halibut, snapper, grouper, mahi mahi, or sea bass.

4 oz/100 g cooked white fish, flaked and bones removed

2 oz/50 g carrot, peeled and cut into chunks

2 oz/50 g sweet potato, peeled and cut into chunks

1 tbsp finely chopped fresh tarragon

2 tsp horseradish sauce

1 oz/25 g polenta

5 oz/125 g herb salad

1 tbsp raspberry vinaigrette (see the wild rice salad recipe on *p136*)

1 Preheat the oven to 350° F/180° C. Meanwhile, boil or steam the carrots and parsnips until tender.

2 Mash the carrots and parsnips, then stir in the flaked fish, tarragon, and horseradish sauce. Adjust the seasoning, then shape the mixture into two small fishcakes.

3 Spread the polenta out on a dinner plate, then gently press the fishcakes in it until they're evenly coated.

4 Place the fishcakes on a lightly oiled baking dish and bake in the preheated oven for 20 minutes, or until heated through.

5 Put the herb salad in a bowl, add the raspberry vinaigrette, and toss.

6 Transfer the salad to a dinner plate. Arrange the fishcakes on top and serve immediately.

broiled fish with sweet potato and spinach bake

③ protein ② carbs ③ fat ① saturated fat

200 g/8 oz white fish, such as halibut, snapper, grouper, or sea bass.

200 g/8 oz sweet potato, peeled and cut in half

150 g/6 oz fresh spinach, well washed

50 g/2 oz light sour cream

1 whole nutmeg

1 Preheat the oven to 350° F/180° C. Meanwhile, parboil the sweet potato for 5 minutes, then drain. Allow to cool, then cut into thin slices.

2 Place the spinach in a pan of boiling water for 30 seconds to wilt it. Drain immediately.

3 Put a third of the spinach in the bottom of a small pyrex dish. Grate about ⅓ tsp nutmeg over it, then spread about a third of the sour cream on top. Now, add a layer of sliced sweet potato, using about one-third of the pieces.

4 Repeat the process twice, ending with a layer of sweet potato on top.

5 Place on the top shelf of the preheated oven and bake for 35 minutes, or until completely cooked.

6 About 10 minutes before the sweet potato and spinach bake is due to be ready, preheat the broiler and cook the fish until done to your liking.

7 Take the bake from the oven and spoon it onto a dinner plate. Lay the fish alongside, season to taste, and serve immediately.

polenta-crusted swordfish with sweet potato

③ protein ② carbs ② fat ⓪ saturated fat

6 oz/150 g swordfish or other meaty fish (salmon, tuna, or cod)

6 oz/150 g sweet potato, peeled and cut into cubes

1 oz/25 g polenta

for the marinade

½ pint/300 ml skim milk

2 tbsp finely chopped fresh tarragon

1 Make the marinade by mixing the milk and tarragon in a bowl.

2 Place the fish in a flat-bottomed dish, cover with the marinade and leave to marinate for at least an hour. (For best results, cover the dish with plastic wrap and leave it in the fridge overnight.)

3 Preheat the oven to 350° F/180° C. Meanwhile, spread the polenta out on a dinner plate. Season it with salt and pepper. Remove the fish from the marinade and then gently press it in the polenta until it's evenly coated.

4 Seal the outside of the fish by cooking it for 2 minutes on each side in a hot, dry skillet. Transfer it to a lightly oiled baking dish and bake it in the oven for a further 8 minutes, or until golden and cooked through.

5 Meanwhile, boil the sweet potato until soft, then mash.

6 Spoon the mashed sweet potato onto a dinner plate and lay the cooked fish on top. Season to taste and serve.

marinated tuna with polenta

② protein ③ carbs ③ fat ① saturated fat

For maximum flavor – and to cut down on preparation time the day of making – I generally start marinating the tuna the night before. And on warm summer evenings, I cook it on the barbecue – it tastes every bit as delicious.

6oz/150g fresh tuna

2oz/50g polenta

12fl oz/350ml skim milk

a handful of fresh basil leaves

for the marinade

2 tsp sesame oil

1 tbsp peeled and sliced fresh root ginger

1 tsp freshly squeezed lime juice

2 tsp soy sauce

3 tbsp water

½ tsp crushed garlic

1 Make the marinade by placing the ingredients in a flat-bottomed dish slightly larger than the piece of tuna and whisking them together.

2 Place the tuna in the marinade and turn it over a few times until evenly coated. Cover the dish with plastic wrap and place it in the fridge for at least an hour (but the longer you leave it the better – overnight is absolutely ideal).

3 Preheat the broiler to hot. Remove the tuna from the marinade, and broil it for about 2 minutes on each side if you like it pink, or 4 minutes on each side if you like it well done.

4 While the tuna is cooking, prepare the polenta – it takes only a couple of minutes. Pour the milk into a saucepan and heat until warm but not boiling. Meanwhile, tear the basil into strips. Stirring constantly, sprinkle in the polenta and basil and cook for a couple of minutes until the polenta is the consistency of mashed potato. Remove immediately from the heat.

5 Spoon the polenta onto a dinner plate. Lay the tuna alongside. Season to taste and serve.

nutrition key

⓪ negligible or none

① low

② medium

③ high

steamed fish with Moroccan vegetables

② protein ③ carbs ② fat ⓪ saturated fat

6 oz/150 g firm white fish, such as halibut, snapper, grouper, mahi mahi, or sea bass

2 oz/50 g pumpkin flesh, cubed

3 oz/75 g sweet potato, peeled and cut into small cubes

2 oz/50 g carrot, peeled and diced

2 oz/50 g zucchini, cut into chunks

2 oz/50 g leek, cleaned and sliced

1 tbsp olive oil

½ tsp cinnamon

½ tsp brown sugar

2 tsp chopped fresh cilantro

2 oz/50 g canned chickpeas (drained weight)

1 tbsp raisins

1 Preheat the oven to 425° F/220° C.

2 Put the pumpkin, sweet potato, and carrot in a pan of boiling water and parboil for 3 minutes. Drain well, and place in a pyrex dish.

3 Mix in the zucchini, leek, olive oil, cinnamon, brown sugar, and cilantro.

4 Place the dish in the oven and bake for 25–30 minutes. Stir once or twice so the ingredients cook evenly.

5 Ten minutes before the vegetables are due to be ready, put the fish on to steam. Five minutes later, add the chickpeas and raisins to the vegetables and mix in well.

6 Spoon the cooked vegetables onto a dinner plate, lay the fish on top, and season to taste.

monkfish with roasted vegetables

③ protein ② carbs ③ fat ① saturated fat

This rather luxurious dish is great for a treat. For less special occasions, you can substitute a piece of any white fish, such as cod, haddock, halibut, or snapper. Ask at the fish counter to have it taken off the bone.

6 oz/150 g monkfish tail, off the bone

3 oz/75 g cauliflower, cut into thick slices

6 asparagus spears, trimmed

4 oz/100 g mushrooms, halved

4 oz/100 g eggplant, cut into chunks

2 slices Parma ham

3 basil leaves

1 tsp capers in brine, drained and chopped

4 black olives, pitted and very finely chopped

2 tsp olive oil

6 fresh rosemary sprigs or 1 tsp dried rosemary

1 Preheat the oven to 400° F/200° C.

2 Lay the slices of Parma ham side by side on a chopping board. Arrange them so they overlap slightly along one edge.

3 Scatter the basil leaves, capers, and olives evenly on top, then place the monkfish on one corner. Roll all the ingredients up so you have a parcel wrapped in Parma ham.

4 Place the parcel in the middle of a large piece of aluminum foil. Wrap the parcel by gathering together the edges of the foil and scrunching them together loosely at the top. Spoon 2 tbsp water in at the top and then seal the parcel up tight, making sure the corners are airtight, too.

5 Spread the olive oil thinly over the bottom of a baking dish. Place the vegetables on top and move them around well so they are all evenly coated. Insert the fresh rosemary sprigs here and there, or sprinkle over the dried rosemary, so the flavor can permeate the whole mixture. Place in the preheated oven.

6 After 5 minutes, place the fish parcel on the baking dish as well.

7 Five minutes later, turn the vegetables so they cook evenly. Leave fish and vegetables to bake for a further 10 minutes.

8 Remove the fish parcel carefully from the foil and place it in the center of a dinner plate. Spoon the vegetables around the outside, season to taste and serve.

smoked salmon and lentil salad

③ protein ③ carbs ② fat ⓪ saturated fat

2 oz/50 g smoked salmon

4 oz/100 g canned green lentils (drained weight)

1 green bell pepper

6 cherry tomatoes

4 oz/100 g arugula

2 tsp freshly grated Parmesan cheese

for the dressing

2 tsp olive oil

1 tsp balsamic vinegar

1 Preheat the oven to 450° F/230° C.

2 Make the dressing by whisking together the olive oil and vinegar.

3 Place the green pepper and cherry tomatoes on a baking dish and bake in the preheated oven for 8–10 minutes, or until they become soft and browned on the outside.

4 Meanwhile, put the arugula leaves, Parmesan cheese, and lentils in a bowl. Drizzle over the dressing and mix together well, so all the ingredients are evenly coated.

5 Take the green pepper and tomatoes out of the oven. Place the pepper in a small plastic bag and loosely tie the neck. Leave for 10–15 minutes, then peel it, cut it in half, and remove the seeds. Slice the flesh into strands and add to the salad.

6 Arrange the cooked tomatoes around the outside of a dinner plate. Place the salad in the middle, and lay the smoked salmon on top. Season with black pepper and serve.

steamed cod with green lentils and tomatoes

③ protein ② carbs ① fat ⓪ saturated fat

Although I'm using cod in this recipe, you could substitute any piece of firm white fish, such as halibut or sea bass. Make sure you ask at the fish counter for any bones and skin to be removed.

6 oz/150 g cod steak

4 oz/100 g canned green lentils (drained weight)

6 cherry tomatoes, skinned

1½ oz/35 g dried porcini mushrooms

2 tsp olive oil

½ red onion, peeled and finely chopped

½ clove garlic, finely minced

1 oz/25 g celery, finely chopped

2 oz/50 g leek, cut into thin strips

1 tsp finely chopped fresh thyme or ½ tsp dried thyme

1 tsp finely chopped fresh parsley

1 Soak the porcini in a small bowl of warm water for about 15 minutes.

2 Put the cod on to steam. Cook for 15–20 minutes depending on the thickness of the fish.

3 While the cod is steaming, heat the olive oil in a skillet. Once the oil is hot, add the finely chopped onion and cook until soft.

4 Add the garlic, celery, and leek and cook for a couple more minutes. At this point, you may need to add a tablespoon or two of hot water to the pan to stop the ingredients sticking.

5 Drain the porcini mushrooms, reserving the water they were soaking in. Chop the mushrooms finely and then add them, along with the water they were soaking in, to the vegetables in the skillet. Cook for a further 2 minutes.

6 Finally, add the lentils, tomatoes, thyme, and parsley, and cook for a further 3 minutes.

7 Spoon the lentil and tomato mixture onto a dinner plate. Lay the steamed cod on top, season to taste, and serve immediately.

nutrition key

⓪ negligible or none

① low

② medium

③ high

lemon shrimp with three bean salad

② protein ③ carbs ② fat ⓪ saturated fat

3 oz/75 g large fresh shrimp, shelled

4 oz/100 g canned black eye beans (drained weight)

2 oz/50 g canned red kidney beans (drained weight)

2 oz/50 g canned chickpeas (drained weight)

½ red bell pepper, thinly sliced

½ yellow bell pepper, thinly sliced

1 tbsp chopped fresh cilantro

2 tsp olive oil

2 tbsp freshly squeezed lemon juice

for the dressing

1 tsp clear honey

2 tsp wine vinegar

½ tsp paprika

1 With a sharp knife, slice down the back of each shrimp. This gives them a better texture for eating. Rinse them in cold running water, then pat dry with a paper towel.

2 Mix the beans and chickpeas in a bowl. Add the peppers and cilantro and stir well.

3 Make the dressing by whisking the ingredients together in a cup, then drizzle it over the salad and toss well.

4 Heat a wok or frying pan and add the olive oil. Add the shrimp, and keep them moving around. Once they start to cook, and the backs open up where you've sliced them, drizzle them with lemon juice and cook a few seconds more.

5 Arrange the salad on a dinner plate. Top with the shrimp, and serve.

wheat-free pasta with tomato and shrimp sauce

③ protein ③ carbs ① fat ⓪ saturated fat

Any pasta made from corn, rice, or maize is suitable for this dish.

6 oz/150 g wheat-free pasta, cooked according to the packet instructions

9 oz/225 g canned chopped tomatoes and their juice

3 oz/75 g cooked shrimp

1 tsp olive oil

1 tsp finely minced garlic

1½ oz/35 g onion, peeled and finely chopped

1½ oz/35 g mushrooms, chopped

1 tbsp red wine (optional)

1 tsp finely chopped fresh oregano or ½ tsp dried oregano

2 tsp finely chopped fresh basil

1 Coat the bottom of a warm frying pan with the olive oil. Add the garlic and onion, and cook until soft.

2 Add the mushrooms, and, if the pan is getting dry, a little water. When the mushrooms are starting to soften, add the red wine (or 1 tbsp water). Let the mixture bubble for a moment, then add the oregano and basil.

3 Now add the tomatoes and juice and stir well so the tomatoes dissolve in the sauce. Finally, add the shrimp and stir well. Turn the heat down and allow to simmer for 15–20 minutes, stirring occasionally. The sauce should reduce to a thick consistency.

4 Place the pasta on a dinner plate, top with the sauce, and season.

wheat-free pasta with turkey

③ protein ③ carbs ② fat ① saturated fat

4 oz/100 g wheat-free pasta, cooked according to the packet instructions

3 oz/75 g lean ground turkey

2 tsp olive oil

1 oz/25 g red onion, peeled and finely chopped

1 clove garlic, finely minced

2 oz/50 g mushrooms, finely chopped

2 oz/50 g celery, finely chopped

2 tbsp red wine (optional)

2 tsp finely chopped fresh thyme or ½ tsp dried thyme

9 oz/225 g canned chopped tomatoes and their juice

1 Heat a frying pan and then add the olive oil. Add the onion and garlic, and cook until soft but not brown. Add the ground turkey and cook, stirring, until lightly browned.

2 Add the mushrooms and celery, then turn the heat down slightly. If necessary, add a little water to the pan to stop the ingredients sticking.

3 When the mushrooms and celery are beginning to soften, add the red wine (or 2 tbsp water) and thyme and stir well. Allow the mixture to bubble for a few moments, then add the tomatoes and their juice and stir.

4 Turn the heat down and leave to simmer, stirring often, for another 12–15 minutes, or until the mixture has reduced to a thick sauce and the turkey is cooked.

5 Place the pasta on a dinner plate, top with the sauce, and season.

chicken with couscous and mint yogurt

② protein ③ carbs ① fat ⓪ saturated fat

3 oz/75 g roasted chicken, skinned and cut into bite-sized pieces

4 oz/100 g couscous

1 oz/25 g black olives, pitted and finely chopped

2 tbsp freshly squeezed lemon juice

a few fresh basil leaves

for the mint yogurt

1 tbsp finely chopped fresh mint

1 oz/25 g cucumber, finely diced

4 tbsp fat-free plain yogurt

1 Prepare the couscous according to the packet instructions. While still warm, mix in the olives and lemon juice. Tear the basil leaves into shreds and add them as well. Stir well.

2 Make the mint yogurt by mixing the mint, cucumber, and yogurt in a small bowl. Season to taste.

3 Spoon the couscous onto a dinner plate, arrange the chicken on top, then dress with the mint yogurt.

marinated chicken with steamed vegetables

③ protein ③ carbs ③ fat ① saturated fat

For maximum flavor, the chicken needs a good hour to marinate before you cook it. If you have the time to prepare it the night before, all the better! As far as vegetables are concerned, use a mixture of whatever you have on hand, or your favorites. Keep experimenting, though, so you find the combination you like most.

1 skinless, boneless chicken breast

14 oz/350 g vegetables (choose from a mixture of carrots, eggplants, green beans, leeks, mushrooms, bell peppers, zucchini, and snow peas)

for the marinade

2 scallions, finely chopped

2 cloves garlic, finely minced

2 tsp peeled and finely minced fresh root ginger

2 tsp paprika

2 tsp ground cumin

1 tbsp freshly squeezed lemon juice

½ pint/300 ml warm water

2 tsp olive oil

a pinch of saffron threads

1 Make the marinade by placing all the ingredients in a flat-bottomed dish and mix them together well so the flavors combine.

2 Slice the chicken breast through the middle so you have two thin filets. Place them in the dish and coat them thoroughly with marinade. Cover the dish with plastic wrap and leave in the refrigerator for at least an hour, and up to 24 hours.

3 Preheat the grill to hot. Remove the chicken from the marinade and grill for about 6 minutes on each side, or until the chicken is cooked all the way through.

4 Meanwhile, put your choice of vegetables on to steam.

5 Arrange the steamed vegetables on a plate. Lay the chicken filets alongside, and season to taste. Serve immediately.

nutrition key

⓪ negligible or none

① low

② medium

③ high

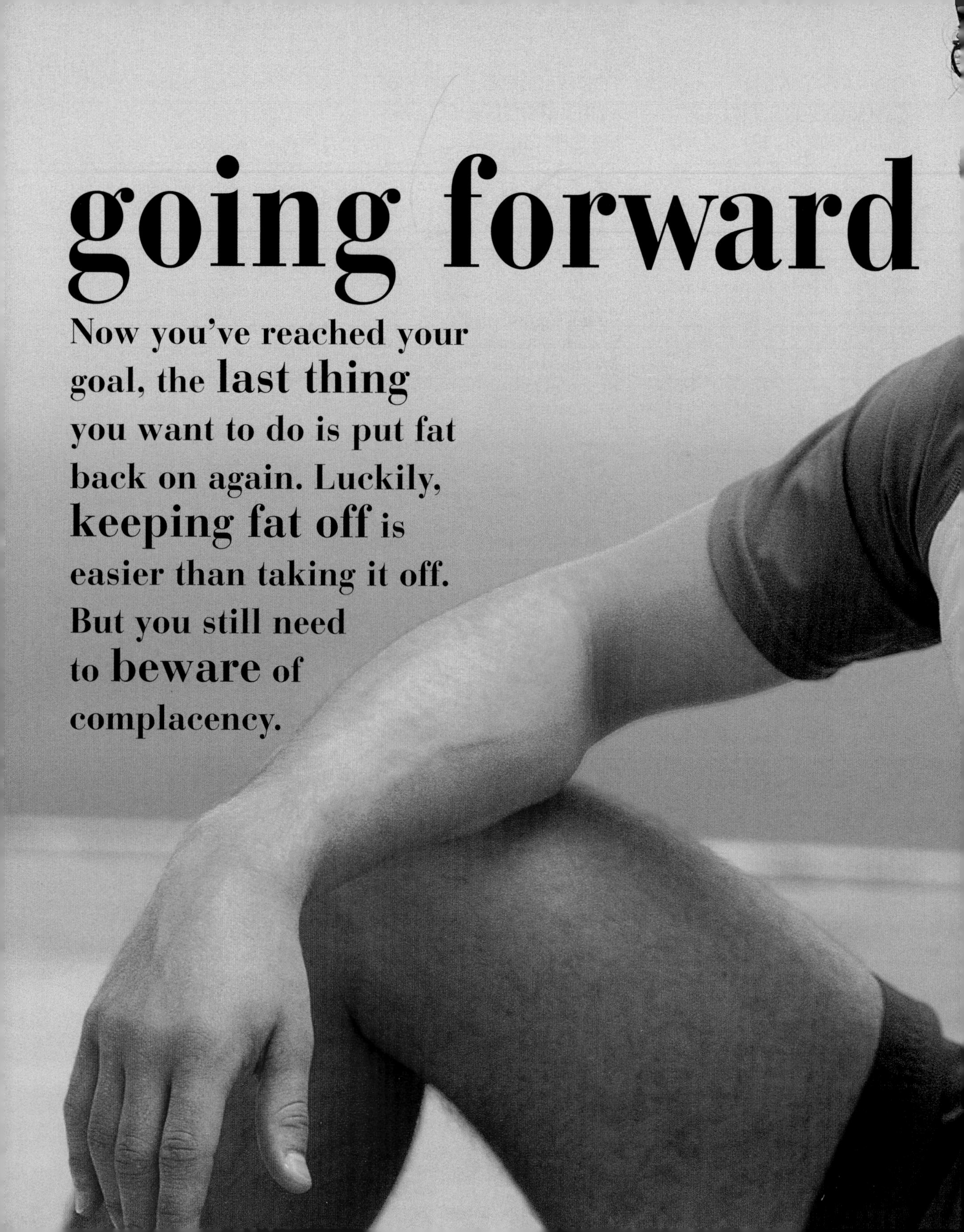

going forward

Now you've reached your goal, the last thing you want to do is put fat back on again. Luckily, keeping fat off is easier than taking it off. But you still need to beware of complacency.